COPING WITH CANCER

Coping with Cancer

Léa K. Jacobs
Editor

Nova Science Publishers, Inc.
New York

For permission to use material from this book please contact us:
Telephone 631-231-7269; Fax 631-231-8175
Web Site: http://www.novapublishers.com

Library of Congress Cataloging-in-Publication Data

Coping with cancer / Léa K. Jacobs, editor.
p. ; cm
Includes bibliographical references and index.
ISBN: 978-1-60456-213-2 (hardcover)
1. Cancer--Psychological aspects. 2. Adjustment (Psychology) 3. Cancer--Nursing. I. Jacobs, Léa K.
[DNLM: 1. Neoplasms—psychology. 2. Adaptation, Psychological. 3. Caregivers—psychology. 4. Quality of Life. 5. Stress, Psychological. QZ 200 C7828 2007]
RC262.C632 2007
616.99'4—dc22

2007048712

Published by Nova Science Publishers, Inc. ≃ *New York*

Contents

Preface		vii
Expert Commentaries		
Commentary A:	The Role of the Breast Cancer Nurse Specialist *Ilana Kadmon*	1
Commentary B:	Use of Linguistics to Promote Coping with Cancer *Erin O. Bantum and Jason E. Owen*	7
Short Communication:	Technologic Innovations that Will Improve the Quality of Care and the Quality of Life for the Cancer Patient *David S. Lester and Michael N. Liebman*	13
Chapter I	Stress and Coping in Caregivers of Pediatric Cancer Survivors *Katherine Conlon Hutchinson and Melanie J. Bonner*	23
Chapter II	Parental Coping with Childhood Cancer *Annika Lindahl Norberg*	61
Chapter III	Toward Psychological Intervention for Cancer Patients: Emotional Suppression, Psychological Distress, and Coping with Cancer *Yumi Iwamitsu and Ross Buck*	77
Chapter IV	Dialogues in Palliative Cancer Care: The Value of Responsive Evaluation to Develop Shared Understandings of Good Care *Tineke A. Abma and Guy A. M. Widdershoven*	95
Chapter V	Can Coping Predict Quality of Life and Survival over a Five-Year Period in Women with Breast Cancer in Anthroposophic and Conventional Care? *Marianne Carlsson*	107
Chapter VI	Cancer as a Family Affair: How the Illness Influences Family Life - a Nursing Science Perspective *Katharina Lex*	127
Index		141

Preface

Millions of people alive today have faced a diagnosis of cancer. Some of them are newly diagnosed or are undergoing treatment. After a diagnosis of cancer, one may feel shock, disbelief, fear, anxiety, guilt, sadness, depression, and anger. Each person may experience some or all of these feelings. People with cancer typically feel the sooner they get rid of the cancer, the better. They may feel rushed to make decisions. People facing cancer often find themselves facing the possibility of their own death. At first, some focus on dying from cancer instead of living with cancer. This new book presents research issues on this topic.

Expert Commentary A – Coping with a diagnosis of breast cancer is a very demanding situation and a great challenge for any woman. Multiple factors may influence this process of coping at various levels. It may be affected by age, family and social support, socio-economic background and even the level of formal education. Moreover, women diagnosed with the disease may have to face many professionals and may have to go through a variety of tests and to confront other issues that may also have an effect on their coping and managing the situation. Lately, women are increasingly involved in the decision-making regarding their care, which may also add to the difficulty related to this period. It is for these reasons that breast care nursing has developed as a profession, with the major objective and aim of helping women and their family members to cope with this challenge (Marks-Manan and Pope, 1985; Rabinowitz, 1987; Henke-Yarbro, 2003; Burnet et al., 2004). In this commentary, the history of breast cancer nursing will be briefly described, as well as the specific meaning of its role in the modern Western world.

Expert Commentary B – Many researchers and clinicians have found that one way to help people cope with cancer is through the facilitation of emotional expression. Emotional expression can be promoted with relative ease in clinical settings and research endeavors. In addition, there are many ways in which researchers and clinicians have measured emotional expression. One of the ways in which researchers have sought to gain information regarding who expresses emotion is through the use of self-report inventories. While this appears to be an obvious way to measure emotional expression there is some concern regarding the accuracy of capturing the actual amount and nature of emotion expressed through the use of self-report measures. Another, and perhaps more accurate way of identifying both the presence and intensity of a range of emotions is through computational linguistics. Interventions promoting the expression of emotion result in a wealth of rich textual data. This data has been found to be a useful tool in predicting for whom and when emotionally expressive driven tasks are useful. Computational linguistics are efficient, although there is room for growth with some of the frequently used programs. These programs as well as ideas for enhancing the current programs will be discussed in the commentary.

Short Communication – From a regulatory perspective, quality of life can be measured based on a series of physical measurements which provide a "quantitative" evaluation of palliation due to a specific treatment, e.g. therapeutic intervention. This is usually evaluated during the performance of a clinical trial under controlled conditions that are aimed at obtaining regulatory approval of a therapeutic entity for a specific indication. Palliation can be determined by two approaches: 1) pain and symptom managements as defined by the World Health Organization as palliative care, and/or) interventions that are non-curative, such as chemotherapy, surgery and/or radiotherapy which all focus on treatment. So, according to the regulatory perspectives, which focus on the institutionalized system of healthcare, the focus is based on management of the disease from the provider, payer, pharmaceutical company, etc. perspectives. This approach dictates the form of treatment that is to be prescribed, often reimbursed, for the patient. This has created a business model where the driver is often the new technology, whether a therapeutic, device, management program, that has received regulatory approval. The question of whether this really provides the best palliative care from a patient perspective is not well-addressed (Petersen, M.A., Pedersen, L, and Groenvold, M. Palliat.Med., 2007, 21:289).

This commentary will focus on innovative approaches that will directly impact and potentially improve the care for the cancer patient from a patient's perspective. If we are to look at the present healthcare approach, each technological intervention is considered to be THE "iPod", while in reality it is the patient who should be considered the "iPod" and all of the interventions are the "accessories" that the patient would require in order to manage their disease. Is there going to be a day where the patient will choose which "accessories" they would like to utilize to manage their disease, an equivalent to "iTunes"? This article will focus on some of the available "accessories" that could be chosen by the patient or provided by the healthcare service either as a choice or as required, resulting in cancer being to some degree a "designer" disease in terms of management. Considering the potentially terminal nature of cancer, perhaps the patient should have a greater say in their personal management?

From a patient perspective, there are five major stages in pre- and post-management of the disease where technologies can be integrated: starting with pre-symptomatic detection and extending to post intervention, Risk, Diagnostics and/or Early Detection, Intervention, Adherence, and Control. Each of these will be dealt with separately and examples and expected impacts will be provided.

Chapter I – As the new population of pediatric cancer survivors and their families grows, there is increased need for psychosocial research on adjustment and its predictors. Indeed, parents of pediatric cancer survivors often face residual effects of the disease and its treatment, plus the risk of newly emerging late effects or disease recurrence, that require significant long term follow up and care. Parental stress and distress have been shown to be ongoing, suggesting that parents continue to struggle with adapting to the "new normal" and have ongoing fears about the long term health and wellbeing of their child. The objective of this chapter is to identify salient intervention targets to reduce caregiver stress in parents of pediatric cancer survivors. First, the authors will review Thompson and Gustafson's transactional stress and coping model as a framework for understanding the maternal mediational processes involved in adaptation to chronic illness, particularly as it relates to parents of pediatric cancer survivors. This model focuses on the adaptational processes, namely stress appraisal, coping response and family functioning, which contribute over and above the contributions of illness and demographic parameters. These variables may be appropriate intervention targets to reduce, and perhaps prevent, the caregiver stress experienced by parents of pediatric cancer survivors. Then the authors will provide an in depth review of the multidimensional sources of stress facing this population using parents of children with learning disabilities as a comparison group to inform their study of parental stress and coping in parents of pediatric cancer survivors. They will conclude that parents of cancer survivors are a chronically stressed population critically in need of intervention. Finally, the authors will propose that interventions designed to target chronic stress in parents of learning disabled children are a rich source of data to inform the design and implementation of interventions for parents of pediatric cancer survivors.

Chapter II – Cancer in a child alters the life situation of the family. For the parents, it implies stressors of varying duration, predictability, and impact. In addition to concerns about the child's prospects of being cured from cancer, the strain relates to, for example, witnessing the child in pain, concerns about the child's future, the quality of care, supporting siblings of the ill child, negative employment and financial consequences, accepting the intensity of one's own reactions, and dealing with the reactions of others. Eventually, some parents must face the death of their child. Nonetheless, successfully completing treatment does not automatically imply a "happy end", since impairments due to aggressive cancer therapies, as well as to the illness itself, are relatively common. All in all, this combination of stressors, ranging from minor hassles to traumatic experiences, places a considerable burden on parents.

Through the trajectory of childhood cancer, the varying contexts of stressors sketched out above activate various psychological processes. Accordingly, the disclosure of the diagnosis of childhood cancer implies a psychological and existential challenge for a parent. Immediately after being informed of the child's cancer diagnosis, even successfully adjusting parents experience arousal, sleep disturbances, and other symptoms of severe stress. Furthermore, several events activate stress responses during cancer treatment. In addition, long-lasting and accumulating stressors can lead to the psychological and physical exhaustion of chronic stress. Once treatment is completed, the tangible as well as the existential aspects of everyday life need to be re-established. Moreover, parents who lose their child will be subject to grief that for a period dominates life.

Permanent psychiatric problems are rarely seen in parents of children with cancer. Nevertheless, even temporary stress can have negative effects for the parents themselves and for their children. Thus, many parents are likely to benefit from professional support interventions, brought into line with the specific psychological processes involved. This chapter outlines parental stressors, demands, challenges and burdens of childhood cancer, exemplifying the processes that may follow.

Chapter III – Most patients facing cancer experience strong negative emotion including depression, anxiety, and sadness. They have worries including fear of death, fear of cancer, recurrence of cancer, and side-effects of treatment. Moreover, they worry about their family, their job, and their quality of life. In particular, patients who demonstrate the Type C behavior pattern including emotional suppression, and those who show higher anxious preoccupation, fatalistic and helplessness/hopelessness attitudes to cancer tend to manifest higher psychological distress. On the other hand, those who show a fighting spirit to cancer tend to experience lower psychological distress. Therefore, coping patterns under extreme stress are key factors predicting psychological distress and QOL. The authors' research has suggested that certain coping patterns including emotional suppression is associated with psychological distress before and after disclosure of cancer. Therefore, the authors proposed that patients need effective psychological intervention immediately after disclosure of the cancer diagnosis. In addition, it is important for patients to continue these interventions during the progress of treatment. The critical aspects of these psychological interventions include encouraging the expression of emotion, inducing fighting spirit, accepting negative emotions, learning how to communicate their emotion appropriately, to encourage better coping with cancer and to decrease psychological distress. In this paper the authors introduce their method and initial trial study of psychological intervention.

Chapter IV – Responsive evaluation is a methodology in which stakeholders assess the value of care in ongoing dialogues in order to create mutual understandings and to improve the quality of care. In this chapter, the authors illustrate the usefulness of a particular genre of responsive evaluation, in which stories and dialogues are central. Stories – for example about the relationships between cancer patients and nurses or between family caregivers and nurses – can illuminate the meaning of everyday situations and experiences. If evaluators listen to the stories of stakeholders, and foster dialogues about these stories among groups of stakeholders, the mutual understanding and respect between the parties will enhance, and shared actions for quality improvements in care may evolve. The authors will show how this approach in palliative care for cancer patients can help to foster conversations about controversial issues such as resuscitation policy, patient autonomy and needs of family caregivers. Through dialogues answers to ethical questions can become shared understandings about good care, leading to joint actions to improve care.

Chapter V - A great deal of research concerning understanding of psychological distress in women with breast cancer has been conducted within the theoretical model of stress and coping. Ways of coping with stress are often classified into two major categories: problem-focused and emotion-focused. Quality of life is a multidimensional concept that refers to a person's perceived quality of her/his physical, psychological, social and existential functioning. Quality of life could be looked upon as an outcome of coping. The aim of the study was to study the relation between coping, quality of life and survival in two samples of women with breast cancer. Another aim was to study the stability of ways of coping over time and whether it would be possible to predict quality of life and survival at a later time from coping at a specific time. The women (n =120) took part in a longitudinal study of the outcome of anthroposophic and conventional care over a five-year period. Sixty women who had chosen anthroposophic hospital and 60 individually matched women from an outpatient department with conventional care participated.

Coping was measured by the Mental Adjustment to Cancer scale and quality of life by the functional scales of the EORTC QLQ-C30 and the Life Satisfaction Questionnaire.

The women were categorised into four categories based on their MAC-scores at inclusion. The categories were called: low copers, high copers, emotional copers and fighters.

Data were collected at six times, at inclusion to the study, after 1 month, after 3 months, after 6 months, after 1 year and after 5 years. Data were collected from 1995 to 2005.

There were differences in perceived quality of life between women with different ways of coping at admission to the study. The women categorised as fighters assessed higher quality of life compared to the other women and also in comparison with Swedish women in general. There was no relation between cancer stage, time since diagnosis and ways of coping. The women in anthroposophic care as well as the women in conventional care showed the same pattern over time, emotional copers assessed lower quality of life compared to fighters and high copers. Most women changed their way of coping and that was more obvious among the women who were treated within anthroposophic care. There was no relation found between ways of coping and cancer stage, time since diagnosis, or survival.

Chapter VI – In Germany, every Year some 425,000 people are newly diagnosed with cancer. About 217,000 people of them will die [1]. Not only is the patient suddenly confronted with enormous stress. As the majority of the German population is surrounded by "relevant other people"- family, friends, colleagues, neighbours etc.- many more people than those having been diagnosed suffer from the cancer [2, 3, 4, 5]. In this chapter the author shall give an overview over the areas of family life which might be affected by the illness. After an introduction the author shall comment on the new family concept and discuss effects on partnerships, children and communication patterns within families. The author shall then examine family coping strategies and responsibilities for nurses. In my conclusion the author aims to show some of the challenges for the nursing profession working with cancer patients.

In: Coping with Cancer
Editor: Léa K. Jacobs, pp.1-5

ISBN: 978-1-60456-213-2

Expert Commentary A

The Role of the Breast Cancer Nurse Specialist

Ilana Kadmon
Hadassah Medical Organization, Jerusalem, Israel

Coping with a diagnosis of breast cancer is a very demanding situation and a great challenge for any woman. Multiple factors may influence this process of coping at various levels. It may be affected by age, family and social support, socio-economic background and even the level of formal education. Moreover, women diagnosed with the disease may have to face many professionals and may have to go through a variety of tests and to confront other issues that may also have an effect on their coping and managing the situation. Lately, women are increasingly involved in the decision-making regarding their care, which may also add to the difficulty related to this period. It is for these reasons that breast care nursing has developed as a profession, with the major objective and aim of helping women and their family members to cope with this challenge (Marks-Manan and Pope, 1985; Rabinowitz, 1987; Henke-Yarbro, 2003; Burnet et al., 2004). In this commentary, the history of breast cancer nursing will be briefly described, as well as the specific meaning of its role in the modern Western world.

Breast Care Nursing as a specialty goes back a quarter of a century to the early 1980's. Some of the first reports about the role of the breast cancer nurse and its importance in supporting and counseling women with breast cancer originated from the UK (e.g. Maguire et al., 1980a; Denton, 1888; Watson et al., 1988; Denton, 1991). Maguire and his colleagues, as far back as 1980, described in their article entitled "Planning a Caring Programme" the importance of monitoring the psychosocial well-being of women with breast cancer, and the significance of the role of the nurse counselor in providing such a service. Denton (1996), a pioneer in implementing such a position, wrote one of the first books on breast cancer nursing, in which she describes the many aspect of the role of the nurse, including information giving, providing counseling, advice, emotional support and follow-up (Denton, 1996). In an article in 1991, she already described the issue of a commitment to quality care (Denton, 1991). It is no more just a role of supporting and helping women diagnosed with breast cancer, she writes, but the role must have some influence on the quality of care of women confronted with the disease. Fallowfield, together with colleagues, in a series of articles along the 1990's, also discussed and demonstrated the importance of counseling cancer patients in general, and women with breast cancer in particular (Fallowfield, 1988; Roberts and Fallowfield, 1990; Fallowfield, 1991; Fallowfield and Roberts, 1992).

These reports from the UK have affected other Western countries such as the US, Australia and Scandinavia (White, 1998; Wilkes et al., 1999; Hordern, 2000). In Australia, Wilkes and colleagues (1999) carried out research (both qualitative and quantitative) to examine how the support needs of women with breast cancer were met. They looked at this issue both from the nurses' and the patients' perspective. This study is an example of a close examination of the newly developed role of the breast care nurse in Australia. Parle and colleagues (2001), also in Australia, examined the rate of detection of psychological morbidity in women by the specialist breast nurses. They discovered that detection was low and that referral to psychosocial services was consequently lacking.

Other studies tried to evaluate the role of the breast care nurse by some objective measures. Such attempts included studies that aimed at demonstrating the importance of the role in reducing women's levels of anxiety and distress and helping them to deal with the diagnosis and consequent treatment. Some studies have shown that women who had the benefit of being followed and counseled by a specialist nurse, dedicated and trained to do so, did better in most psychosocial tests which measure psychiatric morbidity such as the Hospital Anxiety and Depression Scale and other specific mood scales (e.g.Maguire et al., 1980b; Watson et al., 1988; Fallowfield, 1988).

Nowadays, it is well established that State of the Art care of women diagnosed with breast cancer is to be provided within a multi disciplinary comprehensive breast cancer center (Eusoma, 2000; Schuster and Whitney, 2000; Chang 2001). The role of the nurse as coordinating and working in the center of such a team is being recognized and moreover researched. Such roles as informally leading the team, ensuring coordination of care, supporting and supplying information to women, are just a few that have been mentioned (Amir, Scully and Borrill, 2004: Gyldenvang, Goldsmith-Mertz and Ankerson, 2005). In addition, advocating and being "the voice of women" in the system has been also at the core of the nurse specialist's work. Many breast care nurses see themselves, first and before everything else, as patients' advocates (Ganz, 1995; Ambler, 1999; Amir, Scully and Borrill, 2004).

The British Association for Surgical Oncology (BASO) produced guidelines for the treatment of symptomatic breast disease (BASO, 2005). In its guidelines the Association mentions the importance of the care of women by a multidisciplinary team and the role of the breast care nurse in that team. The guidelines states that: "The Breast Care Nurse is a part of the breast care team and should be available for all patients undergoing treatment for breast disease. The Breast Care Nurse should be present_particularly at the time of diagnosis and when options for treatment are discussed." (BASO, 2005, p.S3). However, the British organization Breast Cancer Care and the Royal College of Nursing (Breast Cancer Care and the Royal College of Nursing, 2004) express their concern that there are not enough Breast Care Nurses to follow such guidelines and that most nurses state that they do not have enough time to care for the growing number of women diagnosed with breast cancer and to provide them with the basic psychological support. These organizations conclude, in a press release on that topic, that: "We must make sure their role (of the breast care nurses) is developed with appropriate resources and support to ensure that the UK has sufficient breast care nurses in place to care for people with breast cancer in the future". This, of course, is true not just for the UK but for all countries that have started to employ nurses in such a position.

It is interesting to note, that the North American literature does not refer to the role of the breast cancer nurse. However, the Clinical Nurse Specialist's (CNS) role has been around and is well established there for many years. This role includes within it a much wider set of responsibilities and activities than those related to caring for the women and their families. These include: clinical expert, resource person, consultant, educator, change agent, researcher and advocate (Miller, 1995).Other roles in nursing that were defined, especially in the US, are the Nurse Practitioner and the Advanced Practice Nurse (APN). Pennery (2003), a breast care nurse from the UK, discussed all these terms and the newly developed role of the CNS in the UK. She stated that "The term Advanced Nurse Practitioner (APN) is now widely accepted as an umbrella title that encompasses within it the roles of both Clinical Nurse Specialist (CNS) and Nurse Practitioner (NP)".(Pennery, 2003, p. 344).

In Israel, breast cancer nursing as a recognized profession developed, with the generous support of the Israel Cancer Association, since 1996. The first position was established at the Hadassah Medical Organization in Jerusalem. Since then, most of the medical institutions in the country have decided to provide a nurse (and some have two) who will be dedicated to the care of women with breast cancer. To date, there are about twenty five nurses in such a position nationwide. The role in its definition took some elements from the American Clinical Nurse Specialist and from the more traditional British Breast Care Nurse. This group of Israeli nurses defines themselves as Nurse Coordinators, emphasizing the coordination of care for women with breast cancer. Several of the nurses work in the diagnostic clinic, others in the oncology setting, and some follow women along all stages of the disease. Nurses come from various professional backgrounds and experiences and have different formal education in nursing in general, and in breast cancer in particular (Kadmon, 2006).

How specialist nurses help women in coping with the disease is a question that still needs to be further researched. .It seems that their role is fundamental in helping women to adjust to the new and stressful situation. This help includes providing information, giving emotional support,_coordinating the care and referral to other health care professionals when needed. This model of care has now been widely recognized in many Western countries and has also been applied to other health care situations. Judith Stewart, a Breast Care Specialist Nurse in the UK, wrote in an article to Nursing Standard in 2000: "Through supportive counseling, the specialist nurse helps Jane (a patient she describes, *IK*) cope with her grief reactions, body image change and the impact on her sexuality. The support of a breast care nurse meant Jane had a longstanding and supportive relationship during and following her illness" (Stewart, 2000, p. 61).

In concluding, it should be acknowledged that breast cancer nursing (under whatever title it may employ) has a pivotal role in helping women and their dear ones go through the very demanding and stressful situation. A diagnosis of breast cancer means confronting a life-threatening disease. This may have an effect on many aspects of life and therefore has a crucial impact on the consequent quality of life. Increasing women's quality of life, and supporting them in the process of coping with the illness and its related treatment, is the main focus of nursing in the area of breast cancer care

References

Amir Z. Scully J. and Borrill C. (2004) The professional role of breast cancer nurses in multi-disciplinary breast cancer care teams, *European Journal of Oncology Nursing,* 8, 306-314.

Ambler N. Rumsey N. Harcourt D. Cawthorn S. and Barker J. (1999) specialist nurse counselor interventions at the time of diagnosis of breast cancer: comparing 'advocacy' with a conventional approach, *Journal of Advanced Nursing,* 20(2), 445-453.

BASO (2005) Guidelines for the Management of symptomatic Breast Disease, *European Journal of Surgical Oncology,* 31, S1-S31.

Breast Cancer Care and the Royal College of Nursing Press Release (2004) http://www.rcn.org.uk/news/display.php?ID=1335 and area=Press

Burnet K. Chapman D. Wishart G. and Purushotham A. (2004) Nurse Specialists in breast care: developing role, *Nursing Standard,* 18(5), 38-42.

Chang J. (2001) The impact of a multidisciplinary breast cancer center on recommendations for patient management, *Cancer,* 91(7), 1231-1237.

Denton S. (1988) The Role of the Nurse Counsellor, in: Baum M. (ed.) *Breast Cancer – the Facts,* Oxford University Press, Oxford, 96-103.

Denton S. (1991) A commitment to quality care, *Nursing Standard,* 6(10), 50.

Denton S. (1996) *Breast Cancer Nursing,* Chapman and Hall, London/

EUSOMA (2000) The requirements of a specialist breast unit, *European Journal of Cancer,* 36, 2288-2293.

Fallowfield L. (1988) Counselling for patients with cancer, *British Medical Journal,* 297, 727-728.

Fallowfield L. (1991) Counselling and communication in oncology, *British Journal of Cancer,* 68, 481-482.

Fallowfield L. and Roberts R. (1992) Cancer counseling in the United Kingdom, *Psychology and Health,*6, 107-117.

Gyldenvang H. Goldsmith-Mertz B. and Ankerson L. (2005) Quality management – improving the clinical pathway for breast cancer patients, *European Journal of Oncology Nursing,* 9, 79-82.

Henke Yarbro C. (2003) International nursing and breast cancer, *The Breast Journal,* 9(2), 98-100.

Hordern A. (2000) The emerging role of the breast cancer nurse in Australia, *Cancer Nursing,* 23(2), 122-127.

Ganz P. (1995) Advocating for women with breast cancer, *CA Cancer Journal for Clinicians,* 45, 114-126.

Kadmon, I. (2006). A Network of Breast Care Nurses,. In: BAMAH - *Journal for health professionals in the field of cancer,* Published by the Israel Cancer Association. Givatayim. 81-82. (Hebrew)

Maguire P. Tait A. Brooke M. and Sellwood R. (1980)a Planning a caring programme, *Nursing Mirror,* 17th Jan. 1980, 35-37.

Maguire P. Tait A. Brooke M. and Sellwood R. (1980)b Effect of counseling on psychiatric morbidity associated with mastectomy, *British Medical Journal,* 29th Nov. 1989, 1454-1455.

Marks-Manan D. and Pope B. (1985) Breast Cancer Nursing and counseling, *Blackwell Scientific Pub., Oxford.*

Miller, S. (1995) The Clinical Nurse Specialist – a way forward? *Journal of Advanced Nursing,* 22, 494-501.

Parle M. Gallagher J. Gray C. Akers G. and Liebert B. (2001) From evidence to practice: factors affecting the specialist breast nurse's detection of psychological morbidity in women with breast cancer, *Psychooncology,* 10, 503-510.

Pennery, E. (2003) The differing roles of specialist nurses,. in: Harmer, V. *Breast Cancer: Nursing Care and Management,* Wiley Pub., London, 2003.

Rabinowitz B. (1987) Our many roles in working with women with breast cancer, *Plastic Surgical Nursing,* 7(4), 120.

Roberts R. and Fallowfield L. (1990) *The goals of cancer counsellors,* Counselling, Aug. 1990, 88-91.

Schuster T. and Whitney T. (2000) *Multidisciplinary care for patients with breast cancer, Surgical Clinics of North America,* 80(2), 505-533.

Stuart J. (2000) In the supportive role, *Nursing Standard,* 15(2), 61.

Watson M. Denton S. Baum M. and Greer S. (1988) Counselling breast cancer patients: a specialist nurse service, *Counslling Psychology Quarterly,* 1(1), 25-34.

White K. and Wilkes I. (!998) Describing the role of the breast nurse in Australia, *European Journal of Oncology Nursing,* 2(2), 89-98.

Wilkes L. Beale B. Cole R. and Tracy S. (1999) Supportive care for women with breast cancer: Australian nurses' perspective, *Nursing and Health Sciences,* 1, 71-76.

In: Coping with Cancer
Editor: Léa K. Jacobs, pp. 7-11
ISBN: 978-1-60456-213-2

Expert Commentary B

Use of Linguistics to Promote Coping with Cancer

Erin O. Bantum and Jason E. Owen
Loma Linda University, Loma Linda, CA

Introduction

Many researchers and clinicians have found that one way to help people cope with cancer is through the facilitation of emotional expression. Emotional expression can be promoted with relative ease in clinical settings and research endeavors. In addition, there are many ways in which researchers and clinicians have measured emotional expression. One of the ways in which researchers have sought to gain information regarding who expresses emotion is through the use of self-report inventories. While this appears to be an obvious way to measure emotional expression there is some concern regarding the accuracy of capturing the actual amount and nature of emotion expressed through the use of self-report measures. Another, and perhaps more accurate way of identifying both the presence and intensity of a range of emotions is through computational linguistics. Interventions promoting the expression of emotion result in a wealth of rich textual data. This data has been found to be a useful tool in predicting for whom and when emotionally expressive driven tasks are useful. Computational linguistics are efficient, although there is room for growth with some of the frequently used programs. These programs as well as ideas for enhancing the current programs will be discussed in the commentary.

Coping with Cancer

Two of the leading researchers in coping theory and research, Lazarus and Folkman (1980, 1984), have suggested that we are prompted to cope when our goals are threatened, lost, or harmed. A diagnosis and treatment for cancer can be thought of as a threat to many of our goals or intentions regarding how life will progress. Although numerous theoretical constructs have been suggested and incorporated into models of coping, traditionally coping has been thought of as taking place by the use of problem or emotion-focused strategies (Folkman and Lazarus, 1984; Lazarus and Folkman, 1980). While both emotion and problem-focused coping strategies can be helpful and harmful, there are distinct differences between behaviors engaged in to represent problem and emotion-focused coping. Problem-focused coping involves activities that are directly geared towards attending to a given problem, such as scheduling all necessary appointments with your physician. It has been suggested that the goal of emotion-focused coping is to reduce distress (Folkman and Lazarus, 1980) and regulate emotions, which in turn can alter behavior (e.g., seeking emotional support).

Coping by Expressing Emotion

When looking specifically at a cancer population, researchers and clinicians have suggested that coping with cancer through expressing emotion is beneficial for cancer patients (Austenfeld and Stanton, 2004; Stanton, Danoff-Burg, Cameron, Bishop, Collins, Sworowski, and Twillmen, 2000; Stanton, Dannoff-Burg, and Huggins, 2002). While this idea provides information that could readily be incorporated into both a research protocol and clinical intervention, much of the data collected on emotional expression has been accomplished through the use of self-report measures (de Moor et al., 2002; Stanton, Danoff-Burg, Cameron, Bishop, Collins, Sworowski, and Twillmen, 2000; Stanton, Danoff-Burg, and Huggins, 2002). Self-report measures are quick and provide useful information, although there are some drawbacks and questions to be raised about the use of such measures.

Researchers have suggested that the most used measures for assessing emotion-focused coping contain many items that are arguably measuring differing constructs. For example, the COPE is a measure commonly used to assess emotion-focused coping with cancer patients (Carver, Sheier and Weintraub, 1989). With this measure items such as "I get upset and let my emotions out" and "I act as though it hasn't even happened" are constructed as measures of emotion-focused coping. While we know that emotion-focused coping is theorized as leading to both beneficial and harmful outcomes, it is important to elucidate and then highlight those types of expression that are beneficial and those that are either not beneficial or may in fact be harmful. By using a total score from a measure such as this it is unclear as to how these different types of emotion-focused coping are related to outcomes. Blanket statements as a result of findings on a measure that is intended to capture a broad range of emotion-focused coping strategies could not only be inaccurate but could lead to promotion of strategies that may be ineffective or worse harmful. In addition, self-report measures are by definition subjective in nature and rely on the person being assessed to provide an unbiased report. While providing accurate information is most likely the intention of most people answering a self-report inventory, it is not always possible for one to provide unbiased information (Bowman et al., 1997; O'Leary et al., 2007). In addition, self-report measures of emotional expression have not been highly correlated with more objective measures of emotional expression (Owen, Giese-Davis, Cordova, Kroenenwetter, Golant, and Spiegel,

2005), suggesting that there is a disconnect between objective and subjective measures of emotional expression. Researchers and clinicians should be mindful when assuming that outcomes from these measures translate into real-world behaviors.

Textual data is a potentially more objective measure of emotional expression and provides a much fuller perspective of functioning. It provides numerous data points to observe and gives the researcher or clinician a picture of how an individual is coping with diagnosis and treatment. In addition to the fact that text from psychosocial interventions is an objective source from which it is possible to abstract details regarding emotion-focused coping, it is also readily available. Because emotional expression has been fairly consistently linked with beneficial outcomes (2005 meta-analysis), there are many different types of interventions that have been used to promote emotional expression. Some examples include unstructured journaling for women with breast cancer (Smith, Anderson-Hanley, Langrock, and Compas, 2005), online support groups (Lieberman and Goldstein, 2006), and face-to-face support groups (Graves et al., 2003). All of these interventions have potential to provide large amounts of text data to be analyzed.

Analyzing Text for Emotion

In analyzing this type of data manual coding is one method that could ensure an accurate assessment of emotion. This generally involves reading through the text on a word-by-word basis to identify emotion (e.g., Bantum and Owen, in preparation). Creating rules for coding emotion and then establishing reliability with the method is imperative. Manual coding of emotion provides a rich look at how an individual is coping, although it is quite a laborious process. Computational linguistics are an area of study that is not often associated with psychology, although this emerging field has potential to change the way the assessment of emotional expression takes place. Computational linguistics is a broad field of study in which the overarching goal is to study language and computers. Looking more specifically at emotions and computers a sub discipline called affective computing has arisen (Picard, 1998). The study of affective computing involves making developments with computers so that they can recognize and analyze emotion. This field is fairly sophisticated and progress has been made for computers to recognize facial expressions of emotion or identify emotion from speech, sometimes being called affective computers (Picard, 1998).

In regards to computer programs that code text for emotional expression, the Linguistic Inquiry and Word Count (LIWC) is a computer program created by Pennebaker and colleagues (Pennebaker, Francis, and Booth, 2001) to analyze text on a word-by-word basis. While this program was designed to assess for many different dimensions of written text, emotional expression is one of the aspects measured. LIWC has been widely used to assess for emotional expression within a cancer population (i.e., Laccetti, 2007; Smith et al., 2005; Owen et al., 2005), although the program does not take context into consideration. In doing so, there are many times when LIWC over identifies emotional expression (Bantum and Owen, in preparation). Programs such as LIWC have the advantage over manual coding methods of being more time efficient. In a preliminary analysis it appears that while LIWC captures most of the emotional expression present, there is the tendency for it to assume a word is indicative of emotional expression more often than is the case (Bantum and Owen, in preparation).

It is possible that there are aspects of sophistication that could be adapted from other areas of computational linguistics. Word disambiguation is one important area of possible sophistication. Word disambiguation involves recognizing how the same word used in different contexts has different meanings (Picard, 1996). For example, the word merry might typically mean to be happy or cheerful, although used as a noun (e.g., "We rode the merry-go-round.") it does not depict any type of emotional expression. By programming rules or guidelines into a textual analysis program to account for how different parts of speech might be used in cases where there is versus is not emotion being expressed could add a valuable level of accuracy to programs being used in social sciences for emotion identification in text. Key-word-in-context is another method in which keywords are identified along with the context that they are in (Weik, 1996). Processes such as these could provide a more efficient way of coding emotional expression than manual coding while providing additional accuracy to the existing programs.

Conclusion

When presented with a diagnosis of cancer, individuals are challenged to cope with both the diagnosis and treatment. While there are many helpful and unhelpful ways to cope, some research has fairly consistently demonstrated that when individuals cope with their emotions by expressing, instead of suppressing them they are more likely to have better physical and psychological outcomes. Encouraging individuals to express their emotions has been the focus of many clinical research studies and this type of research produces large amounts of text that provide a window into numerous aspects of functioning, including coping. Computational linguistics is a field that has not been truly integrated into the study of psychology, although gains made in this field could readily be incorporated in to working systems for more accurate measurement of emotional expression. Finding a way to use computational linguistics to better understand how people express emotions and under what conditions and what types of emotions are helpful to express could be an extremely fruitful endeavor in both clinical and research domains.

References

Austenfeld, J. and Stanton, A.L. (2004). Coping through emotional approach: A new look at emotion, coping, and health-related outcomes. *Journal of Personality, 72*(6), 1335-1363.

Bantum, E.O., and Owen, J.E. (in preparation). Evaluating the validity of content analysis programs for identification of emotional expression in cancer narratives.

Bowman, J.A., Sanson-Fisher, R., and Redman, S. (1997). The accuracy of self-reported pap smear utilization. *Social Science Medicine, 44*(7), 969-976.

de Moor, C., Sterner, J., Hall, M., Warneke, C., Gilani, Z., Amato, R., and Cohen, L. (2002). A pilot study of the effects of expressive writing on psychological and behavioral adjustment in patients enrolled in a phase II trial of vaccine therapy for metastatic renal cell carcinoma. *Health Psychology, 21*(6), 615-619.

Folkman, S. and Lazarus, R.S. (1980). An analysis of coping in a middle-aged community sample. *Journal of Health and Social Behavior, 21*, 219-239.

Graves, K.D., Carter, C.L., Anderson, E.S., and Winett, R.A. (2003). Quality of life pilot intervention for breast cancer patients: Use of social cognitive theory. *Palliative Supportive Care, 1*(2), 121-134.

Lazarus, R.S. and Folkman, S. (1984). *Stress, Appraisal, and Coping.* New York: Springer.

Lieberman, M. and Goldstein, B. (2006). Not all negative emotions are equal: The role of emotional expression in online support groups for women with breast cancer. *Psychooncology, 15*(2), 160-168.

O'Leary, T.E., Diller, L., and Recklotus, C.L. (2007). The effects of response bias on self-reorted quality of life among childhood cancer survivors. *Quality of Life Research, 16*(7), 1211-1220.

Owen, J.E., Giese-Davis, J., Cordova, D., Kronenwetter, C., Golant, M., and Spiegel, D. (2006). Self-report and linguistic indicators of emotional expression in narratives as predictors of adjustment to cancer. *Journal of Behavioral Medicine, 29*(4), 335-345.

Ortony, A., Clore, G., and Collins, A. (1988). *The Cognitive Structure of Emotions.* Melbourne, Australia: Cambridge University Press.

Pennebaker, J.W., Francis, M.E., and Booth, R.J. (2001). *Linguistic Inquiry and Word Count: LIWC 2001.* Mahwah, NJ: Earlbaum Publishers.

Picard, R. (1998). *Affective Computing.* Cambridge, Massachusetts: The MIT Press.

Smith, S., Anderson-Hanley, C., Langrock, A., and Compas, B. (2005). The effects of journaling for women with newly diagnosed breast cancer. *Psycho-Oncology, 14*, 1075-1082.

Stanton, A., Danoff-Burg, S., Sworowski, L., Collins, C., Branstetter, A., Rodrigues-Hanley, A., Kirk, S., and Austenfeld, J. (2002). Randomized, controlled trial of written emotional expression and benefit finding in breast cancer patients. *Journal of Clinical Oncology, 20*, 4160-4168.

Stanton, A., Kirk, S., Cameron, C., and Danoff-Burg, S. (2000). Coping through emotional approach: Scale construction and validation. *Journal of Personality and Social Psychology, 78*(2), 1150-1169.

Weik, M. (1996). *Communications Standard Dictionary* (Third ed.). New York: Chapman and Hall.

In: Coping with Cancer
Editor: Léa K. Jacobs, pp. 13-21

ISBN: 978-1-60456-213-2

Short Communication

Technologic Innovations that Will Improve the Quality of Care and the Quality of Life for the Cancer Patient

***David S. Lester*[*1] *and Michael N. Liebman*[2]**
[1]Gene Express, Inc., Toledo, OH; President, ITHW, Inc.
[2]Windber Research Institute, Windber, PA; President, Strategic Medicine, Inc.

Introduction

From a regulatory perspective, quality of life can be measured based on a series of physical measurements which provide a "quantitative" evaluation of palliation due to a specific treatment, e.g. therapeutic intervention. This is usually evaluated during the performance of a clinical trial under controlled conditions that are aimed at obtaining regulatory approval of a therapeutic entity for a specific indication. Palliation can be determined by two approaches: 1) pain and symptom managements as defined by the World Health Organization as palliative care, and/or) interventions that are non-curative, such as chemotherapy, surgery and/or radiotherapy which all focus on treatment. So, according to the regulatory perspectives, which focus on the institutionalized system of healthcare, the focus is based on management of the disease from the provider, payer, pharmaceutical company, etc. perspectives. This approach dictates the form of treatment that is to be prescribed, often reimbursed, for the patient. This has created a business model where the driver is often the new technology, whether a therapeutic, device, management program, that has received regulatory approval. The question of whether this really provides the best palliative care from a patient perspective is not well-addressed (Petersen, M.A., Pedersen, L, and Groenvold, M. Palliat.Med., 2007, 21:289).

This commentary will focus on innovative approaches that will directly impact and potentially improve the care for the cancer patient from a patient's perspective. If we are to

[*] Dr. David Lester; 1 Deborah Dr. Morristown, NJ 07960; Email: dlester@geneexpressinc.com; Tel: 973-786-1066

look at the present healthcare approach, each technological intervention is considered to be THE "iPod", while in reality it is the patient who should be considered the "iPod" and all of the interventions are the "accessories" that the patient would require in order to manage their disease. Is there going to be a day where the patient will choose which "accessories" they would like to utilize to manage their disease, an equivalent to "iTunes"? This article will focus on some of the available "accessories" that could be chosen by the patient or provided by the healthcare service either as a choice or as required, resulting in cancer being to some degree a "designer" disease in terms of management. Considering the potentially terminal nature of cancer, perhaps the patient should have a greater say in their personal management?

From a patient perspective, there are five major stages in pre- and post-management of the disease where technologies can be integrated: starting with pre-symptomatic detection and extending to post intervention, Risk, Diagnostics and/or Early Detection, Intervention, Adherence, and Control. Each of these will be dealt with separately and examples and expected impacts will be provided.

Risk

Perhaps one of the most confusing issues that patients face today is the concept of risk. It is probably not any consolation that this is also a troublesome concept for many physicians. The issues revolve around the fact that risk is typically constructed on the basis of population statistics and then is applied to a specific individual, the patient who is sitting before the physician in the office with questions to be addressed. Risk evaluation may utilize clinical measurements on the patient, family history, molecular (e.g. genetic) evaluation, etc or a combination of these factors. Risk assessment typically involves the use of an algorithm (i.e. equation) that integrates these factors within an equation and produces a numerical or logistic response, i.e. 50% risk or high/medium/low risk. The problems that result for the physician and patient include: 1) what does a 50% risk mean to me? 2) How should I(we) respond to this evaluation? 3) What are the options to choose from? 4) Can I ignore this number? 5) Are there even any options that have been shown to work? (e.g. radical mastectomy for BRCA1 mutation carriers in breast disease vs. alternative medicine approaches); 6) If my risk is greater 50%, does that mean I will definitely get the disease? 7) Is there anything I can do to modify my risk? (e.g. diet, exercise, medication) 8) Are there other tests that I should undergo? 9) What have other patients done in my situation and has it worked? From a patient's perspective, some of these issues are being dealt with using social networking sites on the internet (www.patientslikeme.com) , where the patient can gain insights from other people's experiences. But how this relates to the specific individual is uncertain.

These are some examples of the questions and issues raised when attempting to deal with the concept of risk in patient care, both from the physician's and from the patient's perspective. An alternative for consideration involves removing the stigma of risk by converting its direct delivery into an element in designing a truly "personalized health management" plan. In this manner, the focus of the interaction between physician and patient is on the positive planning and implementation of a screening and surveillance program, integrated with a lifestyle, exercise and diet program, that will consider the aspects of risk without directly assigning an individual to be high or low risk. This may be a critical evolution step for personalized healthcare to consider as it is equally problematic when a patient is assigned to either a high-risk category for which no treatment/intervention is easily defined or a low-risk category in which a patient may become complacent and non-compliant with recommended screening, etc. In such cases, it a "new" role for the internal medicine specialist or general practitioner would be that of a "coach", similar to the physician role more than 40 years ago when there wasn't the challenging diversity of interventions available for treatment of the diseased state.

Diagnostics/Early Detection

A diagnostic test is one component in the early diagnosis of a disease. It can give an indication of the nature of the disease (e.g. which tumor type), the state of disease (e.g. metastatic), and can also determine the specific population that should be exposed to a particular treatment. Thus, based on our present management of cancer, there are three particular stages when a diagnostic may be required. One is as a prognostic for risk assessment which provides an estimation of the potential or probability for an individual developing cancer at some stage of their life. In this application it is a predictor and may lead to potential actions that one can take to keep the probability factor as low as possible. The second stage generally occurs because thereis some indication that a person may have developed or possibly could develop cancer based on some signs and symptoms characteristic to specific tumors. In this case, the diagnostic needs to help stratify both the patient and the disease. The third stage is in monitoring a patient's response to treatment and/or recurrence of the initial disease post-treatment (this may not fit the classical description of a diagnostic).

A. Prognostics and Risk Assessment

A prognostic indicator requires evaluation of a variety of factors. These include demographics, including locale (e.g. exposure to toxins, radiation, etc.) and lifestyle (e.g. exposure to sun, eating habits, economic status, etc.). When incorporated with factors such as family history, this begins to develop what may be referred to as the "persona" of that individual. This could be developed as a first "diagnostic screen" and individuals scored so as to determine if further more expensive and possibly invasive prognostics be used as a follow up to make a solid diagnostic prediction of the person's probability to develop cancer.

As a follow up, some tests have been applied and others are being further developed. For example, whole body computer tomography (CT) scanning is provided at a cost to individuals who may consider they have higher risk. These have been supplied as isolated tests or as part of what is called "Executive Health Checkups". The FDA has stated:

> "At this time the FDA knows of no data demonstrating that whole-body CT screening is effective in detecting any particular disease early enough for the disease to be managed, treated, or cured and advantageously spare a person at least some of the

detriment associated with serious illness or premature death." (http://www.fda.gov/cdrh/ct/).

This does not mean that this test is not necessary but rather that there is insufficient data to make solid conclusions that this sort of prognostic really provides value. In addition, there are many genetic tests that are being developed which will be available also at Executive Health Centers and if deemed appropriate based on a provider request. However, at the level of the provider there seems to be limited acceptance or use of such tests in a prognostic manner. This may be due to their limited understanding of the value of the tests, subsequently how to utilize this to the patient's benefit and the issue of reimbursement of the cost of such tests. As noted above, these is also the potential for negatively impacting the patient and their quality of life when characterization of "high risk" does not have an obvious prevention or intervention associated with it. From a healthcare perspective, there is limited reimbursement of such tests, even though some payers are beginning to recognize their significance by having guidelines such as Aetna and Horizon Blue Cross Blue Shield, but it is clear that the pathway is still unclear. In terms of the patients, new services are beginning to emerge such as those provided by 23andMe (www.23andMe) and Navigenics (www.navigenics.com) where the consumer would directly submit their samples for analysis at a fixed fee and the results would be "translated" into a manner which would the end user could apply to their lifestyles so as to reduce the probability factor.

It is important to note that the advent of easy access to technology for measuring gene expression levels has complicated rather than simplified the prognostic testing of patients because of the limited direct linkage of mechanisms of action to observed (e.g. correlated) changes in gene levels or presence of gene mutations. Even BRCA1 and BRCA2, both associated with increased "risk" for breast cancer, are not absolute predictors of disease, and outside of careful watch and wait procedures, only prophylactic mastectomy appears to be associated with minimizing disease potential. The ability to develop a profile for an individual from their genetic make-up, i.e. genome sequence, will remain a goal of molecular research for some time but not become mainstream within the foreseeable future.

B. Diagnostics

Personalized medicine takes information on a patient's genotype or level of gene expression and their clinical data in order to select an intervention that will be used to treat or prevent disease. It provides patient-specific management resulting in greater accuracy, efficacy, safety and speed. A most recent report from the Department of Health and Human Services can be found at http://www.hhs.gov/myhealthcare/news/index.html#Report. Personalized medicine is and will continue to have a significant impact on the cancer patient. The most-cited example was shown in relation to cancer, the case of Herceptin and Gleevec

Herceptin is frequently heralded as a pharmaceutical testimony to pharmcogenomics because of the regulated need to exhibit over-expression of Her2/neu to support prescribing this antibody treatment for breast cancer. The reality is more complex and reflects the problems that face physicians and patients in choosing the appropriate treatment, using the correct clinical tests and understanding and interpreting reports in the public press. Overexpression of Her2/neu can be measured by two different clinically approved tests with only 25% of all breast cancer patients exhibiting the necessary overexpression of the target for Herceptin. Although most patients receive only one of these tests, where both tests have been administered, there is the observation that in 25% of those patients, the tests do not produce the same result. In addition, even with a positive test result, only 40% of the patients will respond to Herceptin treatment. Thus there are approximately 10% of all breast cancer patients for whom Herceptin is of great value and 90% for whom it may not be the right drug, including one group who may be overtreated and one who may be undertreated because of the limitations of the approved testing methods. Neither of these groups is being appropriately managed by use of the approved diagnostics.

In addition to genomic diagnostics, there are rapidly advancing approaches utilizing biomedical imaging being used for diagnosis. Up until recently, identification of tumors and subsequent determination of the impact of intervention were done using Computer Tomography (CT) – scanning. Advances in imaging technologies have dramatically improved the sensitivity of detection and the characteristics of tumors as well as the response to interventions (see http://imaging.cancer.gov/). The application of CT, Magnetic Resonance Imaging (MRI), ultrasound (USG) and Positron Emission Tomography (PET) have all had significant impacts. The latest imaging approach is using the combined PET-CT scanners which provide high resolution functional data overlaid on exquisite anatomical detail. Unfortunately, the availability of many of these newly emerging technologies are limited as they are expensive and require extensive validation in order to provide true community access.

C. Closing Comments on Diagnostics

There is much talk that the introduction of new technologies will raise the cost of healthcare. While in the short term, the start up phase, there needs to be financial outlay and upfront costs, this intelligent investment will result in the development of validated and standardized tools that will provide the opportunity of moving into the “disease prevention” space and ultimately into the “keeping healthy” area. However, there is a misconception in terms of new technologies. The continued rising cost of healthcare is due to a variety of factors, only one of which is new medical technologies. An excellent overview of how changes in medical technologies can impact health care costs can be found at http://www.kff.org/insurance/snapshot/chcm030807oth.cfm. There is general agreement that by moving to prevention directed healthcare system will significantly reduce the major expenditures in health care, including hospitalization and complications and co morbidity factors.

Intervention

A. Regulated Products

i) Therapeutics

We constantly hear of the continual increased costs of development of new drugs. Estimations are now well over $1 billion to just get a drug to market, which still does not guarantee commercial success. In addition, there are increasing regulatory pressures, including new FDA reforms (http://www.forbes.com/2007/09/21/drugs-safety-fda-biz-sci-cx_mh_0924fda.html?partner=biotech_newsletter). All these factors make the present business model of the "blockbuster" drug, impractical. In addition, there is a continued push for personalized medicine (see Diagnostics) which is also creating the demand for a new business model for therapeutic intervention. This is a very challenging environment but still there remains a strong push with occasional successes for development of new chemical and biologic therapeutic interventions. Because of the difficulty in obtaining a New Drug Approval by the FDA for all drugs, it is not unusual to see already approved drugs receiving approval for new indications. Much of the advance in identification of new therapeutic targets is based on research that is being performed at biomedical research institutions around the world. There is rapid recognition of new potential targets for novel strategies in terms of therapeutic strategies, but there is considerable lag time from identification of targets to development of therapeutics ranging from 7 to 13 years. Excellent insights into the drug development industry can be found at the Tufts Center for Study of Drug Development site (http://csdd.tufts.edu/Default.asp).

ii) Devices

New approaches to targeting tumors are being developed. One of the most intriguing approaches is the targeted therapy. Biomedical imaging is being used to target therapy or tissue resection. Therapy can be either pharmaceutical or some form of targeted radiation treatment. Some of these targeted therapies may use "vehicles" to carry the therapy to the target tumor rather than acting directly upon the desired target. The advantage of this approach is that it is hoped that the adverse events will be limited due to localization of the treatment and also ensuring that the dosage is specifically targeting the tumor ensuring maximal efficacy. Numerous different types of carrier vehicles are being developed, including lipid particles and metallic spheres.

iii) Alternative practices

Because of the spread of information by the internet, there is a growing interest in alternative treatments, including remedies and treatments to offset side effects of chemotherapy and radiation treatments. There are many informative and reliable sites (e.g. http://www.cancer-info.com/alt-ther.htm). However, there is limited scientific data at the level of pharmaceutical and device treatments including well controlled trials. None of these alternatives have undergone stringent regulatory requirements, but this is not to say that they don't have benefit. The potential benefit is based upon personal experiences of others. This is a growing area and as patients gain more and better information on these alternative remedies, it will have a greater impact on the total patient care management of the cancer patient and survivor.

Adherence

Up until recently, the term "compliance" was used to describe patient persistence in taking prescribed medication. This has been "softened" and the terms "adherence" is preferred. In relation to adherence, it is astonishing that persistence of medication of drugs such as Gleevec is not 100%. A recent report at the ASCO 2006 annual meeting showed that numbers with chronic myelogenous leukemia and gastrointestinal stromal tumor (the two tumor types indicated for Gleevec therapy), 25 -30% of patients were not taking prescribed dosages. This could result in lower plasma levels which would significantly reduce the efficacy of the drug. In addition, the drug does not eradicate the disease so it is essential to maintain therapy according to physician directions which is both costly and has adverse effects. Thus, patient support programs and physician communications are critical. There has been an explosion of social networking groups on the internet which provide opportunities for all relevant persons to give personalized feedback and guidance to the patient. This developing technology is extremely addictive and is growing in acceptance at an exponential rate. This is demonstrated by the significant increase in such sites. At the recent first Health 2.0 Conference in San Francisco (www.health2con.com), companies such as WeGo Health, Kosmix, Healthline Networks, Patients LikeMe, Sophia's Garden, Inspire, MedHelp International, to name just a few presented on promising search tools as well as social networking sites. The question was raised as to how does the patient determine which information site or source is "trustworthy"? Also, these companies tend to be "fragmenting" the healthcare space, similar to the pharmaceutical and device industry approaches. What is required is a convergence of these various technology pushes as it is the combination of these approaches that will provide the best management for the patient and survivor.

When considering issues such as adherence (or compliance), one should also examine the larger framework in which the physician and patient exist on a daily basis. Studies are underway to evaluate the issues of diversity in terms of disease detection, presentation and response, notably examining the noted differences in breast cancer survival between Caucasian and African American women. The scope of these studies incorporates molecular and clinical characterization of the patient and tumors, but is further exploring the relationships involving socio-economic, cultural, community support, education, physician-interaction, etc to determine where the comprehensive "eco-system" becomes a factor in causing the observed differences and how it can be better managed, if possible.

In addition to these internet based technologies, there are new devices that can be used to remind patients to take their medicine. Some of these approaches are quite creative, for example, providing colored lights as signals (http://www.ambientdevices.com/cat/orb/

orborder.html) and cell phone reminders (http://www.vocel.com). In addition, there are more simplified approaches being used by payers that simply monitor e-prescription filling. This has been extended in some examples to incorporate Radio- Frequency ID tags (RFIDs) to ensure that the patient is taking the right pill at the appropriate time (e.g. http://www.medicom.bang-olufsen.com/sw431.asp).

All of these approaches are to ensure that the patient is using their interventions in the appropriate manner which will limit adverse events as well as ensure that they are taking the correct formulations for maximized efficacy. In order for the intervention to be truly effective, it must become a part of the daily routine for the cancer patient and their family or support group.

Control

By control we mean managing and evaluating the impact of the intervention. There are of course body fluid tests for monitoring safety. In terms of efficacy, CT scans are most commonly used but there are advances in other imaging technologies such as USG and PET which could prove useful. These have increased specificity and sensitivity.

It would be of great value to have standard tests for determining drug levels in order to assure that they are within the range of the therapeutic index for that therapy. One such approach is the development of specific antibodies for ultimate use in standard immunodiagnostic testing (e.g. www.saladax.com). This would have a significant impact on managing adverse events.

An interesting approach is the development of point of care diagnostics. This allows the patient to monitor specific "biomarkers of disease progression" in their home environment. This would be of great benefit as it provides true palliative value. One such system (www.theranos.com) is developing a packaged system that would measure specific biomarkers, possibly the drug and/or its metabolite levels, then transmit wirelessly to a centralized reading site which would then monitor that the dose is within the therapeutic index and not be at levels that raise the chance of adverse events. This is a technological challenge as it requires multiple incremental technologies to all be working together. And assuming that the technology works, it is still unclear of the adoption rate by the various stakeholders including the patients and the physicians. Add on to that the lack of clarity of the payer system in the US or high level of proof demanded by payment advisory committees, and the future success of such technologies in clinical care practice are quite risky.

It should also be noted that while we talk about disease states, we need to evolve this construct into understanding disease processes. All of biology results from the convergence and divergence of biological processes that operate within their unique timeframes, interact across these time elements, and fundamentally define the underlying physiological state of a patient as they exhibit normal and/or abnormal development and physical behaviors. As these technologies continue to evolve to enable high throughput analysis and evaluation of high resolution data from both the clinical and molecular levels, it will become increasingly important to recognize the differences between the processes of disease and the processes of the "host" or patient. Our understanding is likely to evolve to separate these two sets of processes which are simultaneously operational in a patient as a means to enhance our ability to develop the best levels of patient (and disease) management. Could this ultimately lead to a cure rather than a treatment?

Conclusion

There are many innovations in terms of technology that are presently being developed. There seems to be great promise but we must ensure for maximal advantage to be provided to the patient, the focus must be on the value to the patient care and management. It cannot be driven by payers or providers as ultimately quality of life is a very personal measurement. In addition, to achieve maximum benefit for these technologies, it is important that these varied approaches are not seen as one vs. another but rather how can they be combined in order to provide maximal value. The limits of each of these innovations need to be demonstrated and expressed in a manner that the individual cancer patient can make choices that best suit them for both treatment and recovery. This will provide the ultimate palliative value. But the future is very exciting and promising.

In: Coping with Cancer
Editor: Léa K. Jacobs, pp. 23-60

ISBN: 978-1-60456-213-2

Chapter I

Stress and Coping in Caregivers of Pediatric Cancer Survivors

Katherine Conlon Hutchinson[1] and Melanie J. Bonner[2]

[1] Department of Psychology and Neuroscience; Duke University, Durham, NC

[2] Departments of Psychiatry and Surgery; Duke University Medical Center; Department of Psychology and Neuroscience; Duke University, Durham, NC

Abstract

As the new population of pediatric cancer survivors and their families grows, there is increased need for psychosocial research on adjustment and its predictors. Indeed, parents of pediatric cancer survivors often face residual effects of the disease and its treatment, plus the risk of newly emerging late effects or disease recurrence, that require significant long term follow up and care. Parental stress and distress have been shown to be ongoing, suggesting that parents continue to struggle with adapting to the "new normal" and have ongoing fears about the long term health and wellbeing of their child. The objective of this chapter is to identify salient intervention targets to reduce caregiver stress in parents of pediatric cancer survivors. First, we will review Thompson and Gustafson's transactional stress and coping model as a framework for understanding the maternal mediational processes involved in adaptation to chronic illness, particularly as it relates to parents of pediatric cancer survivors. This model focuses on the adaptational processes, namely stress appraisal, coping response and family functioning, which contribute over and above the contributions of illness and demographic parameters. These variables may be appropriate intervention targets to reduce, and perhaps prevent, the caregiver stress experienced by parents of pediatric cancer survivors. Then we will provide an in depth review of the multidimensional sources of stress facing this population using parents of children with learning disabilities as a comparison group to inform our study of parental stress and coping in parents of pediatric cancer survivors. We will conclude that parents of cancer survivors are a chronically stressed population critically in need of intervention. Finally, we will propose that interventions designed to target chronic stress in parents of learning disabled children are a rich source of data to inform the design and implementation of interventions for parents of pediatric cancer survivors.

Introduction

Parenting stress is a fact of life for all parents. Indeed, the parenting role often places demands on parents' resources that require flexibility to adapt. There is a significant amount of variability in both the demands parents face and the resources they have available. Some populations of parents face unique demands that add to the challenge of successful adaptation. Two examples of such populations are parents of children with chronic illnesses and parents of children with disabilities. More specifically, parents of pediatric cancer survivors comprise a new population that face a unique combination of demands, similar in many ways to both parents of children with chronic illness and parents of children with disabilities. Indeed, cure rates for childhood cancer now exceed 75%, up from 30% in 1960 (American Cancer Society, 2007). As this new population of survivors and their families grows, there is increased need to examine the stress and coping processes in these families. As parents serve as primary caregiver and decision maker for their children, parental adaptation to the long term cancer experience impacts the adjustment and quality of life of the cancer survivor and the entire family system.

Survivors of pediatric cancer often face residual effects of the disease and its treatment, plus the risk of newly emerging late effects or disease recurrence, that require significant long term follow up and care. Parental stress and distress have been shown to be ongoing, suggesting that parents continue to struggle with adapting to the "new normal" and have ongoing fears about the long term health and wellbeing of their child (Kazak, Alderfer, Rourke et al., 2004; Van Dongen-Melman et al., 1995; Van Dongen-Melman, Van Zuuren, and Verhulst, 1998). Indeed, parents of pediatric cancer survivors have displayed clinically elevated levels of anxiety up to five years post diagnosis (Wijnberg-Williams, Kamps, Klip, and Hoekstra-Weebers, 2006). In addition to concerns about physical health, pediatric cancer survivors often experience late effects including cognitive and attentional deficits that impact the entire family (Peterson and Drotar, 2006). These concerns, similar to those experienced by parents of children with learning disabilities, require vigilance and action on the part of the parent to identify and meet their child's unique academic and social needs.

In both the chronic illness and disability populations, there is significant variability in the adaptation and adjustment of parents (Dyson, 1996; Van Dongen-Melman et al., 1998). There is some evidence that this variability is not linked directly to child factors, such as severity of illness or disability. Therefore, it is crucial to examine parental variables that may serve to mediate the stress and coping process. The transactional stress and coping model proposed by Thompson and Gustafson (1996) proposes a pathway by which maternal adaptation to stress results from childhood chronic illness. A review of the literature suggests that the maternal mediational processes proposed by the model, namely stress appraisal, coping response and family functioning, may apply to both the cancer survivor and disability populations. Indeed, if this is case, these variables may be appropriate intervention targets for reduction and/or prevention of the caregiver stress experienced by parents of pediatric cancer survivors.

The objective of this chapter is to identify salient intervention targets to reduce caregiver stress in parents of pediatric cancer survivors. We will first review the transactional stress and coping model (R. J. Thompson, Jr. and Gustafson, 1996b) as a framework for understanding the maternal mediational processes involved in adaptation to chronic illness, particularly as it relates to parents of pediatric cancer survivors. Parents of children with learning disabilities serve as a comparison group to inform our study of parental stress and coping in parents of pediatric cancer survivors. We will conclude that parents of cancer survivors experience both common and unique stressors that should be addressed as part of the child's cancer experience. Finally, we will propose that interventions designed to target chronic stress in parents of learning disabled children are a rich source of data to inform the design and implementation of interventions for parents of pediatric cancer survivors.

Caregiver Stress in a Chronic Illness Population

As medical advances in recent decades have improved the survival rates for many childhood illnesses, there has been increased interest in the psychosocial adaptation of both parents and children to childhood chronic illness. Although good adjustment is typical and major psychopathology is the exception, the research on adaptation indicates that childhood chronic illness is a significant life stressor leading to increased risk for psychological adjustment problems (Goldberg, Morris, Simmons, Fowler, and et al., 1990; Kazak and Barakat, 1997; R. J. Thompson, Jr. and Gustafson, 1996a). A significant number of children and parents do develop adjustment problems, and recognition of variability in psychological adjustment has prompted efforts to distinguish the correlates of adjustment that identify individuals at high risk for adjustment problems. The transactional stress and coping model (R. J. Thompson, Jr. and Gustafson, 1996a) of adaptation to chronic illness developed out of prior models of systems-based adaptation that share the common view chronic illness as a potential stressor (Moos and Tsu, 1977; Pless and Pinkerton, 1975). This model recognizes that adjustment is a complex, multi-system process that takes place within a family systems and social-ecological framework (Bronfenbrenner, 1986; Kazak, 1989).

Transactional Stress and Coping Model

Thompson and Gustafson (1996) proposed a transactional stress and coping (TSC) model of adjustment that views chronic illness as a potential stressor to which the individual and family system endeavor to adapt. This model takes into account the role of environmental factors, parenting factors, and child factors in adjustment, and recognizes the bi-directional interactions that take place between factors. Thus, the complex relationship between illness and outcome is not direct. Rather, it is conceptualized to be a function of the transactions among biological, developmental and psychosocial processes, with an emphasis on the maternal and child processes hypothesized to mediate the illness-outcome relationship (R. J.

Thompson, Jr. and Gustafson, 1996a; R. J. Thompson, Jr., Gustafson, Gil, Kinney, and Spock, 1999). The illness parameters in the TSC model reflect illness type and severity and the demographic parameters include gender, age and socioeconomic status. The focus of the model, however, is on the child and maternal adaptational processes that contribute over and above the contributions of illness and demographic parameters.

Development and Validation of the TSC Model

Guided by Lazarus and Folkman's (1984) cognitive model of stress and coping, Thompson and colleagues included three maternal adaptational processes in the basic model: cognitive processes, coping methods, and family functioning. These processes were also selected based on their empirical evidence and salience as potential intervention targets. The specific cognitive processes targeted include appraisal of stress (Lazarus and Folkman, 1984), self-efficacy (Bandura, 1977) and locus of control (Strickland, 1978). Coping methods in the TSC model are categorized as either palliative - a combination of avoidance, wishful thinking and emotional focused coping - or adaptive - problem-focused coping aimed at altering the stressful transaction by attempting to change the environment or self. Family functioning in the TSC model is categorized by three dimensions - conflicted, controlling or supportive - whose utility in predicting psychosocial outcomes in childhood chronic illness populations has been established (Kronenberger and Thompson, 1990). Slightly different adaptational processes are proposed to mediate child adaptation. The hypothesized child adaptational processes include expectations about self-esteem, health locus of control and methods of coping. Support for the mediational effect of these adaptational processes has been found by Thompson and colleagues in a number of cross sectional and longitudinal studies of children with cystic fibrosis and sickle-cell disease.

In a cross sectional study of children with cystic fibrosis (R. J. Thompson, Jr., Gustafson, Hamlett, and Spock, 1992a), the transactional stress and coping model accounted for 39% of the variance in mother-reported internalizing behavior problems, 43% of externalizing behavior problems, and 68% of child-reported symptoms. Demographic and illness parameters accounted for a minority of the variance in child adjustment problems (9-11% and 3-10% respectively). When controlling for demographic and illness variance, child self-worth and maternal anxiety were both found to predict substantial portions of total variance in child behavior problems. Similarly, in a cross sectional study of children with sickle-cell disease (R. J. Thompson, Jr., Gil, Burbach, Keith, and et al., 1993b) the model accounted for 30% of the variance in child-reported symptoms and 45-49% of the variance in mother-reported behavior problems. When controlling for demographic and illness variance, maternal anxiety accounted for 16% and 33% of mother-reported internalizing and externalizing behavior problems, respectively. In addition, children's strategies for coping with the pain associated with sickle cell disease accounted for 20% of the variance in child-reported symptoms.

Subsequent longitudinal studies of the stability and change of child psychological adjustment provide additional support for the model. In particular, for children with cystic fibrosis, child self-worth accounted for 38% of the variance in child reported symptoms, and maternal distress accounted for another 8%. Overall, low levels of child self-worth and higher levels of maternal distress differentiated stable poor from stable good child adjustment (R. J. Thompson, Jr., Gustafson, George, and Spock, 1994). Results from Thompson et al.'s (1994) longitudinal study of children with sickle cell reinforced this connection, in that children's pain coping strategies accounted for significant variance (19%) in child adjustment. However, unlike the cross sectional study, maternal anxiety did not contribute to child adjustment. These results indicate that different variables within the transactional stress and coping model may be salient targets for disease specific interventions.

Thompson and colleagues also examined maternal adjustment in both cystic fibrosis and sickle cell populations. In the cross sectional study of mothers of children with cystic fibrosis (R. J. Thompson, Jr., Gustafson, Hamlett, and Spock, 1992b), 34% of mothers met criteria for poor adjustment on a well-known measure of mental health (SCL-90). Elevations in the clinical range of distress occurred for 21% of mother on the depression subscale and 18% on the anxiety subscale. The variables in the transactional stress and coping model accounted for over half the variance in maternal depression and anxiety symptoms. In contrast, illness and demographic factors accounted for less than fifteen percent. The largest single variable impacting maternal adjustment was daily stress, which accounted for a 30% increment in mother-reported depression and 22% in mother-reported anxiety. In addition to higher daily stress, mothers with poor adjustment had higher levels of use of palliative coping methods, higher levels of family conflict and lower levels of family support.

In a similar study of maternal adjustment in the sickle-cell population (R. J. Thompson, Jr., Gil, Burbach, Keith, and et al., 1993a), over one-third of mothers met criteria for poor adjustment on the SCL-90. The variables in the transactional stress and coping model accounted for over fifty percent of the variation in maternal distress, with the vast majority accounted for by psychosocial and mediational processes. Illness and demographic parameters, however, accounted for less than ten percent of variance in maternal distress. When illness and demographic factors were controlled for, three additional variables accounted for significant increments in the variance: the ratio of palliative to adaptive coping mechanisms (30%), stress of daily hassles (13%) and emphasis of control in family functioning (3%).

Further support for the TSC model was provided by a longitudinal study of the stability and change in the psychological adjustment of mothers of children and adolescents with cystic fibrosis and sickle-cell disease (R. J. Thompson, Jr., Gil, Gustafson, George, and et al., 1994; R. J. Thompson, Jr., Gustafson et al., 1999). Indeed, maternal adjustment classifications were stable over a 2-year assessment period for 56% of cystic fibrosis group and 77% for the sickle-cell disease group. The results indicated that for both groups of mothers, poor adjustment was consistently associated with greater use of palliative coping, higher levels of daily stress, and lower levels of family supportiveness. Of note, child adjustment only contributed to maternal adjustment in the cystic fibrosis group. Mothers of children with cystic fibrosis also reported higher levels of illness-related stress and family conflict, while mothers of children with sickle-cell disease reported a higher palliative coping ratio.

The TSC model has been successfully applied to a variety of childhood chronic illnesses (R. J. Thompson, Jr. and Gustafson, 1996c). Overall, the work of Thompson and colleagues indicates that mothers of chronically ill children demonstrate rates of poor adjustment between 34 and 57 percent, and that adjustment rates vary somewhat across illness groups (Kronenberger and Thompson, 1992; R. J. Thompson, Jr., Gil et al., 1993a; R. J. Thompson, Jr., Gil et al., 1994; R. J. Thompson, Jr., Gustafson et al., 1999; R. J. Thompson, Jr., Gustafson et al., 1992b; R. J. Thompson, Jr., Zeman, Fanurik, and Sirotkin-Roses, 1992). The overall TSC model accounts for one- to two-thirds of the variance in adjustment. Mediational processes account for large portions of variance in maternal adjustment over and above illness and demographic contributions. More specifically, persistently good maternal adjustment is associated with lower levels of stress, less use of palliative coping methods, and higher levels of family supportiveness. Notably, illness severity did not make a substantial contribution to the variance in maternal adjustment.

Maternal adjustment is important because it is has been related to the adjustment of children with chronic illness. In particular, maternal anxiety has accounted for significant variance in mother-reported internalizing and externalizing child behavior problems (R. J. Thompson, Jr., Armstrong et al., 1999; R. J. Thompson, Jr., Gil et al., 1993b). Mothers who consistently rated their children as having behavior problems and poor adjustment have significantly higher rates of self-reported depression, anxiety and overall distress than mothers who rated their children as having good adjustment (R. J. Thompson, Jr., Gustafson et al., 1999), a finding that supports the impact of maternal adjustment on parenting and child well-being. Indeed, Thompson and Gustafson (1996) conclude, "parenting may be the one common pathway through which the influence of the larger social ecological context within which the child is embedded affects his or her development," (pp. 149).

Adaptation of the TSC Model for Childhood Cancer Survivors

Parents of children that have survived treatment for childhood cancer have much in common with parents of children with other chronic illnesses. Clearly, while children are receiving treatment for cancer the potential for elevated levels of stress and anxiety is high. However, evidence indicates that even after completing treatment there are challenges that persist, requiring families to adapt to a new normal state of daily life that includes added social, emotional and financial stress (Van Dongen-Melman et al., 1998). Indeed, studies of survivors have examined many salient potential stressors, including cognitive late effects, social functioning, post-traumatic stress, secondary cancers and endocrine issues (Nagarajan et al., 2003; Oeffinger and Hudson, 2004; Oeffinger et al., 2004; Zebrack et al., 2004). Results of research on parents of cancer survivors to date has yielded conflicting results, with some indicating overall high rates of good adjustment (Frank, Brown, Blount, and Bunke, 2001) while others indicate high levels of persistent distress (Sloper, 2000; Van Dongen-Melman et al., 1998). This variability evokes questions regarding the sources of stress, the measurement of parental adjustment, and the potential mediators of adjustment in this population.

Sources of Stress

Concern about a child's well-being is a stressor for any parent. For parents of cancer survivors, this concern is magnified by the ongoing risks of physical and cognitive late effects and concerns about the child's social and emotional well-being. Parents themselves must adjust emotionally to the role of parenting a cancer survivor, and cope with uncertainty, grief and loss that are unique to the survivor population. Mothers in particular may be at risk for poor adjustment. Indeed, studies of pediatric cancer populations have shown that up to three-quarters of mothers consistently identify themselves as the primary medical caregiver of a pediatric cancer patient/survivor (Bonner et al., 2006).

The ultimate goal of cancer treatment is to eradicate the cancer. Unfortunately, effective treatments often come at a cost to the patients' long term physical and cognitive health. As such, oncologists attempt to maintain a balance between effective therapy and acceptable toxicity. In some cases, high doses of treatments such as chemotherapy and radiation are associated with higher cures rates yet more severe long term sequelae. In contrast, seeking to minimize toxicity may increase the risk of relapse or disease progression (Moore, 2005). Physical health consequences for cancer survivors vary as a function of the specific diagnosis and treatment. Younger age at treatment is generally associated with more severe late effects (Oeffinger and Hudson, 2004). Late effects following chemotherapy differ based on type of chemotherapy, and may include endocrine dysfunction, bladder or kidney disease, cardiomyopathy, osteoporosis, infertility, secondary cancers, hearing loss, and neurocognitive deficits (Oeffinger and Hudson, 2004; Oeffinger et al., 2004).

Moore (2005) proposed a model in which neurocognitive outcomes are predicted by factors such as chemotherapy, radiation and brain injury on brain development. This relationship is mediated by cognitive intervention, medical parameters (e.g., surgical effect and tumor location) and other factors, including gender, age at treatment and elapsed time since treatment. A younger age at treatment and female gender are associated with poorer outcomes, as is the presence of adverse medical events (e.g. meningitis, shunt infections). Brain tumors and leukemia, specifically acute lymphocytic leukemia (ALL), have been the focus of many studies of neurocognitive outcomes in cancer survivors because they have the most profound effect on functioning both directly and indirectly, as a result of treatment of the central nervous system (CNS) (Armstrong and Mulhern, 1999; Moore, 2005). Children with malignant tumors of the brain and central nervous system account for approximately 20% of all childhood cancers diagnoses (Armstrong and Mulhern, 1999; Zebrack et al., 2004), while children with leukemia, cancer of the blood, comprise approximately 30% (Armstrong and Mulhern, 1999; Moore, 2005).

Children with ALL are at high risk for brain metastases, therefore treatment prophylacticly targets the CNS. Traditionally, CNS preventative therapy has included cranial radiation therapy (CRT) and intrathecal methotrexate. Due to the risks of CNS toxicity, however, treatment is now usually limited to intrathecal and systemic chemotherapy, except for those children who present with CNS disease at diagnosis. However, use of intrathecal methotrexate still places children at an elevated high risk for neurocognitive sequelae (Butler and Mulhern, 2005). Indeed, in one recent study, children who completed treatment for moderate risk ALL exhibited significantly poorer performance in tests of attention, memory, and visual construction than controls (Brown et al., 1992). However, Copeland et al. (1996) conclude that, when treated with systemic chemotherapy alone, children with ALL typically exhibit minimal neurocognitive deficits. Use of intrathecal methotrexate appears to predict much of the variability in neurocognitive outcomes for children with ALL. When neurocognitive impairments do occur, they have a significant impact on a child's success in school, self esteem, social relationships, and long term quality of life.

Children who survive malignancies of the brain are at high risk for a complex combination of physical and neurocognitive sequelae. The presence of a brain tumor in and of itself infringes upon brain development. The aggressive therapies used to treat brain tumors place children at even greater risk for severe deficits. In addition to surgical resection of the tumor, chemotherapy with or without cranial or craniospinal irradiation is indicated for malignant tumors (Butler and Mulhern, 2005). In the physical domain, survivors may experience hearing and/or vision loss, growth failure, seizures, endocrine dysfunction, chronic fatigue and gross and fine motor impairments (Armstrong and Mulhern, 1999). In the cognitive domain, survivors experience deficits in memory (Dennis et al., 1991), academic (Armstrong and Mulhern, 1999) and attentional functioning (S. J. Thompson et al., 2001). Rates vary as a function of gender, age at treatment, tumor type, tumor location and treatment type (Butler and Copeland, 2002; Mulhern, Kovnar, Kun, Crisco, and Williams, 1988). Females and children under the age of 4 years that receive radiation therapy, particularly whole-brain radiation, are at highest risk for intellectual decline (Moore, 2005). Although children with brain tumors are a heterogeneous group, they are a distinct and unique subgroup of survivors that are clearly placed at the greatest risk for severe late effects due to the disease and its treatments.

The physical and cognitive late effects exhibited in cancer survivors extend the impact of the disease indefinitely, posing additional and chronic parenting and caregiver stress. Indeed, recent research indicates that parents of learning or cognitively disabled children exhibit higher levels of distress than do parents of nondisabled children (Baker and McCal, 1995; Dyson, 1996; Fuller and Rankin, 1994). For parents of brain tumor and ALL survivors, one source of stress may be related to the academic environment of the survivor. Indeed, a recent review found that reintegration into school settings can impact psychological adjustment and quality of life of survivors and their families, particularly for children surviving cancers of the central nervous system (Peterson and Drotar, 2006). For most survivors, ongoing educational intervention is needed to accommodate the acquired learning disabilities that arise in the years following treatment. For parents, this involves close monitoring of their child's progress, understanding of their unique strengths and weaknesses, working with schools to develop and implement an individualized education plan, understanding state and federal laws and regulations, obtaining appropriate therapy, and considering children's future professional or occupation potential. Parents will need to be informed advocates for their children. This can be a time consuming and difficult task, thereby contributing to already elevated levels of parenting distress that were associated with the diagnosis and treatment of a life-threatening illness.

Impairments in social functioning that are also seen in survivors of cancer additionally may contribute to the difficult task of parenting a survivor (Patenaude and Kupst, 2005). In one study, survivors were described by teacher, peer and self-rating to be more socially isolated than matched controls (Vannatta, Gartstein, Short, and Noll, 1998). Survivors received fewer friendship nominations than controls, and peers viewed the survivors as being sicker, more fatigued and more often absent from school. In addition to frequent absences and physical symptoms, there may be a neurocognitive aspect to cancer survivors' social impairments. Indeed, children treated for brain tumors are at increased risk for acquiring deficits consistent with the nonverbal learning disability syndrome (Buono et al., 1998; Carey, Barakat, Foley, Gyato, and Phillips, 2001). This syndrome is characterized by problems in social perceptions, social judgment and social interaction skills. These effects, which emerge over time, can negatively impact a child's quality of life in both the academic and social realm.

Parents of cancer survivors must also help their children emotionally adjust to life after cancer. Children surviving cancer show considerably variability in their overall adjustment. In one study examining psychological outcomes of brain tumor survivors and their siblings, demographics, socio-economic status and physical health status were found to be associated with distress. Being in poorer health, female, non-white, low-income, unmarried and unemployed were all associated with higher self-reported levels of distress (Zebrack et al., 2004). Although the overall rates of clinical levels of distress were comparable to the general population, brain tumor survivors were more likely to report symptoms of distress than their siblings. This can largely be accounted for by both higher rates of physical health problems and limited opportunities in regard to work, school and marriage among cancer survivors. In addition, although treatment intensity did not directly correlate with psychological well-being, it may be an indirect influence by limiting social opportunities that are directly related to well-being (Zebrack et al., 2004). Given the influence of child well-being on parent well-being, and the extended caregiver role associated with parenting a cancer survivor, elevated levels of distress in survivors may contribute to increased distress in parents of survivors. In addition, if a survivor is not able to work, attend school or marry, they will be more likely to depend on their parents for financial and emotional support, long after what would be expected.

The psychosocial effects of childhood cancer continue into adulthood. One study examined the role of parent-child relationships as a mediator of adult outcomes (Hill, Kondryn, Mackie, McNally, and Eden, 2003). Adult survivors were more likely than controls to have impaired romantic relationships and friendships and poorer day to day coping. The findings also indicate that mothers and fathers have different roles in the transition to adulthood for cancer survivors, with fathers being less encouraging of adult social roles, less critical and less controlling than mothers. Survivor's impaired close relationships were independently associated with lower father encouragement and greater mother involvement, particularly for female survivors. Lower father encouragement was also associated with poor daily coping, particularly for young males. These findings illustrate the impact of parent-child relationships on the attainment of normative adult goals, such as development of close, non-family relationships.

A recent qualitative analysis of strains, resources, and coping behavior in families impacted by childhood cancer illuminated strains caused directly by the cancer and health-care system, as well as those related to the child, family, and community (J. Patterson, Holm, and Gurney, 2004). Cancer and child related strains included secondary illness, disabilities, attentional deficits, and loss of a normal lifestyle and activities. Family strains included strong parent emotions, balancing multiple family needs, such as time for other children and work, and financial strains. Community strains included dealing with the insensitivity or avoidance of others, school issues, and lack of formal support. Despite the children in this sample being, on average, 4 years post-treatment, these issues remained salient sources of distress and considerable strains on the families' resources.

Van Dongen-Melman and colleagues (1995) investigated late psychosocial sequelae in a sample of parents of children who survived cancer and found that childhood cancer had distinct and persistent late psychosocial effects on parents of survivors. Uncertainty and loneliness were the most frequently reported problems. Moderate levels of anxiety, depression and disease-related fears were reported by one third to one half of the respondents. Specific predictors of distress included demographic and situational characteristics such as being a mother, low socio-economic status, no religious affiliation, chronic disease in a family member other than the child surviving cancer, and concurrent stressors. The treatment itself had little or no effect on reported problems. However, when treatment led to long-term sequelae in the child, a significant and specific effect on parental problems was observed. This suggests that it is not the acute stressors during active treatment, but the emergence of new disease-related stressors that impact parent adjustment.

In a follow-up study, Van-Dongen-Melman and colleagues (1998) used qualitative techniques to gain insight into the emotional experiences of parents of childhood cancer survivors. They audio-taped 85 open-ended interviews with mothers and fathers of cancer survivors, and identified a number of salient dimensions on which families showed variability. There were several domains in which parents experienced a sense of loss. Nearly every parent reported a loss of positivity towards life and a sense that they would never again be the same relaxed person they were prior to their child's diagnosis. Many parents also reported a loss of invulnerability for trauma. They described this as fragility in their psychological equilibrium that rendered them less able to cope with stressors. A third loss was that of time and energy that was spent caring for their ill child that could have been spent differently had their child not been ill.

Late effects, whether physical and psychological, of the cancer and its treatment, contribute to parents' sense of loss with respect to the child. Parents in Von Dongen-Melman's sample described the loss of the child they had prior to the cancer. Although their child was considered cured, he or she was not necessarily the same healthy child as before. Some of the children became mentally and/or physically handicapped as a result of their disease, contributing to the loss of the image and reality of a healthy child (Van Dongen-Melman et al., 1998). These reports are consistent with the cumulative findings that parents with disabilities and chronic illness suffer long-term periodic sadness (Burke, Hainsworth, Eakes, and Lindgren, 1992). Indeed, parents report "chronic sorrow and prolonged feelings of loss, grief, disappointment and fear in response to continual losses associated with chronic illness. While this sorrow is appropriate and understandable, considering the many challenges of parenting a chronically ill child, it does not meet criteria of clinical psychopathology, and therefore often goes unrecognized and untreated (Bonner et al., 2006).

Parents also report continuing feelings of uncertainty and anxiety about the recurrence of the disease and/or the appearance of emerging late effects in their child. As a consequence of this, parents tended to perceive their child as especially vulnerable, both in regards to their physical condition and their psychosocial development. Many parents report trying to compensate for the difficult events during treatment by attempting to protect their child from potentially upsetting or stressful events. In Van-Dongen-Melman's (1998) sample, many parents reported placing physical limitations on their child, while setting fewer psychological demands. As the authors point out, this is in contrast to the developmental process in healthy children in which physical demands are reduced with increasing age, whereas psychological demands are increased. The families able to set demands for their children appeared to be the most balanced and had better child outcomes than families unable or unwilling to do so.

Parents of cancer survivors often lack the typical transition to increased autonomy that occurs when a child reaches young adulthood. Indeed, many parents maintain an extended period of active parenting that may include accompanying their child to medical appointments, providing therapy at home, remedial teaching, psychosocial support or financial support (Ressler, Cash, McNeill, Joy, and Rosoff, 2003; Van Dongen-Melman et al., 1998). This extended caregiving role may interfere with both the long term goals and expectations for their future as parents and children. One study of identity in adolescent survivors of childhood cancer (Madan-Swain et al., 2000) found a greater frequency of survivors in the foreclosed identity status than their healthy peers. Adolescent identity formation requires individuation, a process in which one differentiates the self from the parent without totally disconnecting from the family. The foreclosure state of identity formation occurs when one prematurely commits to certain goals, values and beliefs, often internalizing the values of significant adults in their lives. Reaching identity achievement status requires a period of questioning or reflection that may be particularly challenging for cancer survivors who are simultaneously coping with the physical and cognitive sequelae of their illness. Factors associated with the foreclosed identity status include the disease severity, symptoms of post-traumatic stress disorder and family functioning characterized by greater levels of conflict (Madan-Swain et al., 2000). Perhaps by internalizing their parents' belief system that is defined by uncertainty, sorrow and loss, survivors avoid facing the uncertainty of their futures.

Indeed, uncertainty seems to play a large role in the psychological adjustment of parents of cancer survivors. Mishel (1981; 1983; 1988) defines parental uncertainty as an inability to determine meaning relative to illness in a child. Uncertainty in illness has four dimensions: ambiguity about the illness state; lack of information about the illness, its treatment, side effects and management; complexity in what information is known and relationships with care providers; and the unpredictability of a person's prognosis and quality of life. Uncertainty, although inherently neutral, can be appraised as positive or negative. The appraisal process can be influences by numerous factors, including mental health, perceived illness severity and intensity of treatment, social support, and relationship with care providers (Mishel, 1981, 1983, 1988).

A review of the literature on parental uncertainty (Stewart and Mishel, 2000) included eight studies of cancer survivors. Uncertainty in cancer, characterized by not knowing what caused the cancer, not knowing the child's prognosis, and not knowing how late effects will impact their child's future, is related to psychological distress, characterized by anxiety, depression, cognitive disturbances and feelings of helplessness. Cohen (1995) identified seven triggers that cause a heightened level of awareness and uncertainty in families of children suffering from a life-threatening illness. These included routine medical appointments, body variability, keywords, changes in the therapeutic regime, evidence of negative outcomes, new developmental demands, and nighttime. Each trigger presents a set of conditions that can predict an increase in parental distress, many of which are similar to triggers of posttraumatic stress symptoms that commonly occur in parents of cancer survivors. A recent review of parental uncertainty and posttraumatic stress literatures also support a linkage that may be key to developing interventions to support parents of children with serious illnesses (Santacroce, 2003).

Maternal Mediational Processes

In a qualitative study of parents of cancer survivors, some parents reported positive changes in their lives as a result of the cancer experience (Van Dongen-Melman et al., 1998). Some of these changes concerned restructuring their overall life perspective, putting events into perspective and a greater appreciation for day-to-day life. Some parents reported personal growth and some reported improved marital relations and a greater sense of closeness with family. The cancer experience also resulted in a more gratifying relationship with the child for some parents. These findings raise the question of why some parents are seemingly resilient to the intense stress of the cancer experience. Using the TSC model as a framework (R. J. Thompson, Jr. and Gustafson, 1996b), several variables may serve to mediate the outcome of the cancer experience, including parent cognitions, coping and family functioning.

Cognitive Processe

Parent cognitions have been found to affect child development (Miller, 1988). Parents' causal attributions about why their child behaved in a certain way influences parent affective reactions and choice of socialization strategy (Dix, 1993; Dix, Ruble, Grusec, and Nixon, 1986). They reflect parental beliefs about developmental processes and abilities, such as many parents believe children's behavior becomes increasingly intentional with age (Dix et al., 1986). Maternal tendencies to attribute social skills and difficulties to causes within the child rather than external causes are associated with both maternal stress and poor child social adjustment (Rubin, Mills, and Rose-Krasnor, 1989). There is also growing evidence that parent cognitions, and therefore parent-child interactions, are shaped by social ecological factors (Miller, 1988; Rubin et al., 1989), indicating that parental cognitions are one mechanism through which a the larger environment influences child outcomes.

Childhood cancer is associated with a loss of control by which parents have a very limited ability to control or influence events related to the cancer experience. Attitudes towards control, or attributions, played an important role of the overall wellbeing in the qualitative study of parents of cancer survivors (Van Dongen-Melman et al., 1998). Parents with an extreme orientation towards control, either internal or external, experienced more difficulty in adjustment. Van Dongen-Melman and colleagues hypothesized that parents with extreme internal orientation may be so overcome with a sense of personal responsibility that they may suffer from guilt, anxiety and depression. Additionally, those parents with extreme external orientations blamed their environment, leading to feelings of anger and resentment. However, those parents whose appraisals of control were more balanced seemed to be more accepting of reality and experienced less guilt. This balanced perspective of attributions of control is realistic in this situation; parents have limited possibilities to exert direct control.

There is some evidence that attributional style may also influence cognitive development in chronically ill children. Thompson and colleagues (R. J. Thompson, Gustafson, Bonner, and Ware, 2002) studied a group of young children with sickle-cell disease and found that both biomedical risk and parenting risk were associated with poorer cognitive functioning at 24 months of age. Parenting risk in this case was defined as a learned-helplessness attributional style. A helpless attributional style could be detrimental in parenting an ill child, as parents are likely to take a less active role if they do not feel as though they have control. The same study found that parent adjustment was associated with high levels of daily stress, less knowledge about child development, and lower expectations of efficacy.

Stress appraisal can also play a role in adjustment to childhood cancer. McCubbin and colleagues (2002) conducted in depth interviews with parents in 26 families who had a child treated for cancer within the previous three years. They identified resiliency factors that helped the family recover, including changing their appraisal to make the situation more comprehensible, manageable and meaningful. For example, these parents reported improvements in family relationships, a stronger sense of meaning or purpose, and accommodations in perceptions of "what normal is" to include cancer.

The appraisal of uncertainty may also play a role in parental adjustment. Although most of the current research on coping with uncertainty in chronic illness documents the adverse effects of uncertainty on well being, one study conceptualized uncertainty as a dialectic phenomenon of both distress and personal growth (Parry, 2003). The study consisted of 23 interviews with long-term cancer survivors. Survivors' discussions of uncertainty varied greatly in content and context. Some survivors coped very positively with the uncertainty by adopting a live-for-today attitude and accepting what was out of their control. Many viewed uncertainty as a catalyst for a changed outlook and a deeper appreciation of life. Parry (2003) posits that what begins as a coping strategy for dealing with the uncertainty can evolve into a purposeful life outlook that balances the dialectic of uncertainty and certainty. These results suggest that uncertainty may not always be aversive, and that appraisal of uncertainty may be a salient factor in predicting adjustment in both survivors and their parents.

Coping

Coping methods in the TSC model are categorized as either palliative - a combination of avoidance, wishful thinking and emotional focused coping - or adaptive - problem focused coping aimed at altering the stressful transaction by attempting to change the environment or self (R. J. Thompson, Jr. and Gustafson, 1996b). There is strong evidence to suggest that coping processes have significant relations to psychological symptoms, with problem-focused forms of coping, such as planful problem solving, being negatively correlated with symptoms, and emotion-focused coping, such as avoidance, being positively correlated with symptoms (Folkman and Lazarus, 1988; Folkman, Lazarus, Gruen, and DeLongis, 1986).

Families adjusting to the stress of childhood cancer use a variety of coping behaviors. A recent qualitative analysis of coping behavior in families impacted by childhood cancer illustrated that most families use a combination of appraisal-focused, problem-focused and emotion-focused coping behaviors (J. Patterson et al., 2004). These researchers categorized coping strategies such as being positive and maintaining hope, trusting in God and living in the present as appraisal focus coping. Problem-focused strategies included advocating for the child and seeking information, while emotion-focused included crying, hiding feelings and using humor or fun to cope.

There is evidence that mothers and fathers use differing and sometimes complementary coping methods to deal with the diagnosis of childhood cancer (Goldbeck, 2001). In one study, mothers and fathers did not differ in their self-reported quality of life, despite mothers' report of more frequent and more effective coping. No convergence was found in couples coping styles, and in fact, coping dissimilarity in support-seeking and religion was correlated with the improvement of parental quality of life. Dissimilarity in information seeking, however, was correlated with a decrease in the child's quality of life. Clearly, there are situations when divergent coping skills in parents are adaptive, and times when they are not. This phenomenon, perhaps due to the differing roles of mothers and fathers in caring for the family, is important in planning interventions targeting coping in parents of children with cancer.

Several coping-focused interventions have been tested with families dealing with childhood illness, and the results support the differential impact of adaptive and palliative coping on adjustment. The results of a study of the effects of written emotional disclosure with caregivers of children and adolescents with chronic illness failed to find support for their hypothesis that emotional disclosure would positively impact caregivers' moods and physical symptoms (Schwartz and Drotar, 2004). Instead, the experimental group, who wrote about trauma and stress, experienced significantly less positive affect, more negative affect and more physical symptoms following the task than did the control group, who wrote about summer activities. In addition, when compared to the control group, the experimental group showed no long term improvements in mood, distress or health-related quality of life, or caregiver appraisal. This finding is consistent with research in chronic illness populations that shows negative outcomes for emotion-focused coping.

In contrast, a problem-solving skills training intervention has proved beneficial for mothers of children with newly diagnosed cancer (Sahler et al., 2005; Sahler et al., 2002). Indeed, problem-solving therapy (PSST), a cognitive-behavioral intervention, has been shown to be effective in treating negative affectivity (depression, anxiety) for mothers of newly diagnosed pediatric cancer patients. In one study, 92 mothers were randomly assigned to receive PSST or to receive standard psychosocial care. After the 8-week intervention, mothers in the PSST Group had significantly enhanced problem-solving skills and significantly decreased negative affectivity compared with controls. Changes in self-reports of problem-solving behaviors accounted for 40% of the difference in mood scores between the two groups. PSST had the greatest impact on improving constructive problem solving, whereas improvement in mood was most influenced by decreases in dysfunctional problem solving (Sahler et al., 2002). In a longitudinal follow-up study of 430 English- and Spanish-speaking mothers of recently diagnosed patients, similar effects were found immediately after PSST. Furthermore, the data from the 3-month follow-up indicates some benefits of PSST were still evident. In general, efficacy for Spanish-speaking mothers exceeded that for English-speaking mothers, and young, single mothers benefited the most (Sahler et al., 2005). Understanding how coping methods change and evolve over the course of the illness trajectory is the next step in helping families adjust to cancer and cancer survivorship.

In the qualitative study of parents of cancer survivors, reported coping strategies were categorized as avoidance or confrontation (Van Dongen-Melman et al., 1998). Avoidance strategies included drinking alcohol, smoking, distancing oneself, telling oneself not to think about it, focusing on other issues, such as work and hobbies, striving towards normality, and avoiding information about the disease and its long-term consequences. In contrast, confrontation strategies included seeking information about the disease, talking with other parents of children with cancer, talking with medical staff, seeking help and assistance, and accepting the disease and its late effects. The diversity in coping strategies illustrates the variance in the degree of openness of communication about personal feelings. It appears that a moderate ability to express and deal with emotions may be ideal, as parents described as highly emotionally involved, either anxious or angry, had children whose emotional functioning was below the normal range (Van Dongen-Melman et al., 1998).

Family Functioning

Although the experience of illness may bring some families closer together, other families experience disruptions in familial relationships. Family functioning may be a salient factor accounting for the variance in family adaptation to chronic illness. Family functioning in the TSC model is categorized by three dimensions: conflicted, controlling or supportive, whose utility in predicting psychosocial outcomes in childhood chronic illness populations has been well established (Kronenberger and Thompson, 1990). The conflicted factor is characterized by high conflict, low cohesion and low organization, while the controlling factor is characterized by high control, high achievement orientation, and low independence, and the supportive factor is characterized by high cohesion and expressiveness.

Indeed, higher levels of family supportiveness and lower levels of family conflict were associated with behavior problems in chronically ill children. In one study, Thompson and colleagues (R. J. Thompson, Jr., Armstrong et al., 1999) examined family functioning in a sample of children with sickle cell disease (SCD), and found that conflicted family functioning accounted for a significant portion of mother-reported behavior problems. Similarly, in a longitudinal study of children with SCD (R. J. Thompson, Jr. et al., 2003), an increase in behavior problems was only associated with an increase in family conflict, and not by illness or demographic factors. Therefore, maternal appraisal of family conflict may be a risk factor for chronically ill children with behavior problems and a salient intervention target for fostering adaptation. Family functioning may also directly impact maternal stress in chronically ill populations. In one study of mothers of very low birth weight infants, over the course of their infant's first six months, mothers perceived less stress related to the infant but more stress associated with daily hassles and less family support and more conflict (R. J. Thompson, Jr., Oehler, Catlett, and Johndrow, 1993).

There is evidence to support a similar influence of family functioning on adjustment in cancer survivors. One study of adolescent cancer survivors (Rait, Ostroff, Smith, and Cella, 1992) examined both the perceived family functioning of 88 adolescents (aged 12-19 years) who had successfully completed treatment for pediatric cancer and the relationship between family functioning and post-treatment adjustment. Adolescent cancer survivors reported lower levels of family cohesion than the normative sample of healthy adolescents and their families. Higher perceived family cohesion and adaptability was also strongly related to good post-treatment psychological adjustment for the adolescents.

This relationship also exists in parents of children treated for cancer. Streisand and colleagues (Streisand, Kazak, and Tercyak, 2003) examined the relationship of illness-specific parenting stress and family functioning in a sample of 116 parents of children treated for cancer. After controlling for treatment status (on vs. off treatment), they found that parenting stress related to caring for a child with a medical illness was associated with poorer family functioning. Specifically, parents reporting more frequent illness-related stressors, particularly those of an emotional nature, are more likely to also report difficulty with behavioral control within the family. Thus, it appears that a family encountering significant stress is less likely to be able to create and abide by a set of rules governing appropriate behavior. In addition, the total number of stressful situations encountered by parents is associated with the level of affective involvement with the family, indicating that parents responding simultaneously to a large number of stressors would have diminished amount and quality if emotion resources to provide to the entire family.

The most adaptive style of family functioning may vary over the illness trajectory in families of cancer survivors. For example, in research examining sibling adjustment to childhood cancer, high family adaptability is related to more favorable psychological functioning following the cancer diagnosis (Horwitz and Kazak, 1990). Similarly, family resiliency within three years of the end of treatment has been linked to the ability of families to rapidly mobilize and reorganize in response to childhood cancer (McCubbin, Balling, Possin, Frierdich, and Bryne, 2002). At this time, it may be beneficial for the family to adjust to the illness by temporarily changing family structure, rules and relationships as a function of the demands of the illness and the ill child. However, a recent longitudinal study of sibling adjustment (Houtzager et al., 2004) found that high family adaptability over time was associated with poor sibling adjustment, indicating that it may be harmful for family members adjustment when adaptability becomes a chronic state of constantly fluctuating rules and roles. This could have implications for the influence of family functioning on parental adjustment, as it places a demand for flexibility on the parent. It may be ideal for a parent of a child with cancer to be flexible and adaptable while the child is on treatment, and then revert to traditional roles and rules once treatment is complete. This is consistent with Van-Dongen-Melman's (1998) that families able to set demands for their children appeared to be the most balanced and had better child outcomes than families unable or unwilling to do so.

Social Support

One variable not accounted for in the TSC model is social support. Many forms of social support, including that from health care providers, extended family, the community and the workplace have been linked to good adjustment in families dealing with childhood cancer (McCubbin et al., 2002). One recent study examined the relationship between anxiety, seeking social support as a coping strategy, and perceived social support among mothers and fathers of child with successfully completes treatment for cancer (Norberg, Lindbad, and Boman, 2006). For mothers and fathers, a moderate, positive relationship was found between support seeking and perceived support. Although there was a stronger relationship between anxiety and support for mothers, significant relationships between anxiety, support seeking, and perceived support were present for both mothers and fathers. The relationship for support seeking was much weaker than that for perceived support, indicating that parents' subjectively perceived support appears to be more influential on anxiety symptoms than actual support seeking.

Outcomes Related to Maternal Adjustment

Maternal adjustment is often measured by depressive and anxious symptomology. However, given the compelling evidence regarding the impact of parenting stress on parenting health and behavior and child adjustment, the definition of maternal adjustment to chronic illness needs to be expanded to include measures of parenting stress. Greater stress is associated with less optimal parental functioning, family functioning, and parent-child interactions (Crnic and Greenberg, 1990). Indeed, even minor daily stress may cumulatively result in elevated irritability in the parents and aggressiveness in children (G. R. Patterson, 1983). The relationship between child and parenting functioning in families of chronically ill children is well established (Finney and Bonner, 1992). In recent pediatric cancer research, parental distress was shown to have a negative impact on both parent and child functioning (Robinson, Gerhardt, Vannatta, and Noll, 2007). As such, parenting stress is an important component in the evaluation of overall parental adjustment to chronic illness.

As mentioned above, the findings regarding parent adjustment as related to caring for a child with chronic illness are fairly discrepant, with some studies revealing generally good adjustment (Frank et al., 2001), while others indicate high levels of ongoing distress (Sloper, 2000; Van Dongen-Melman et al., 1995). Consequently, some researchers have recently begun to question the methods with which parental adjustment is currently measured (Eiser, 1998; Streisand, Braniecki, Tercyak, and Kazak, 2001). Recently, a new measure of parent adjustment was developed and validated with a group of parents of children with brain tumors (Bonner et al., 2006; Bonner, Hardy, Willard, and Hutchinson, 2007; Bonner, Hardy, Willard, Hutchinson, and Guill, in press). One-hundred and forty-nine parents of cancer survivors were assessed using the 25-item self-report Parent Experience of Child Illness (PECI). An exploratory factor analysis yielded four factors: guilt and worry, emotional resources, unresolved sorrow and anger, and long term uncertainty. Internal reliability was acceptable, and construct validity was evident in positive correlations with established measures. In contrast to other illness specific measures, the PECI focuses on parents' subjective distress and emotional resources that may play a key role in the adjustment to chronic illness. Use of the PECI with families of children and adolescents with chronic illness is recommended in Brown and colleagues' guidebook to evidence-based treatments for chronic illness (Brown, Daly, and Rickel, 2007). Use of these more sensitive measures will be an important step in discerning the emotional experience of parents of cancer survivors and resolving the discrepancy in current research on parent adjustment.

Kazak and colleagues' research on post traumatic stress symptoms (PTSS) and post traumatic stress disorder (PTSD) in parents of cancer survivors (Alderfer, Cnaan, Annunziato, and Kazak, 2005; Brown, Madan-Swain, and Lambert, 2003; Kazak, Alderfer, Rourke et al., 2004) provides additional evidence of distress in this population. PTSS are common in families of childhood cancer survivors. Indeed, parents report more symptomology than former patients, with one study reporting that nearly 30% of mothers met diagnostic criteria for PTSD since their child's diagnosis and nearly 20% of families had at least one parent currently meeting criteria for PTSD (Kazak, Alderfer, Rourke et al., 2004). In fact, the most recent version of the Diagnostic and Statistical Manual of the American Psychiatric Association (DSM IV; 1994) now recognizes that a life threatening illness in the family can precipitate symptoms of PTSD in patients and their parents. Core symptoms of PTSD in cancer survivors and their families include avoidance of the illness experience (e.g. hospitals and clinics), intrusion of the cancer experience into daily activities and in response to minor illness, and hypervigilance. These symptoms persist for parents long after treatment ends (Kazak et al., 1997). The fact that parents report even greater symptomology than the patients themselves has led to the characterization of parents as "second order patients" (Lederber, 1998).

Elevated distress in parents certainly impacts their children's quality of life, both directly and indirectly. Indeed, high maternal distress is associated with greater child emotional and somatic distress in parents of children following a cancer diagnosis (Steele, Dreyer, and Phipps, 2004). Parenting stress may also contribute to physical health outcomes as well. Many studies examining the impact of acute and chronic stress on health have found that increased stress leads to a decrease in immune functioning and an increase risk of infectious disease in healthy individuals (S. Cohen, Doyle, and Skoner, 1999; S. Cohen, Tyrrell, and Smith, 1991; S. Cohen and Williamson, 1991; Herbert and Cohen, 1993; Naliboff et al., 1991). These physical risks have the potential to negatively impact parenting behavior and child outcomes as well.

Caregiver stress and its impact on health and wellbeing have been studied in a variety of populations, including caregivers of Alzheimer patients and parents of children requiring assistance by technology (Kiecolt-Glaser et al., 1987; Kuster, Badr, Chang, Wuerker, and Benjamin, 2004; Thyen, Terres, Yazdgerdi, and Perrin, 1998). Alzheimer caregivers report insufficient time to rest or exercise, poor self-assessment of health, increased rates of depression and anxiety and lowered immune function (Kiecolt-Glaser et al., 1987; Lu and Austrom, 2005). Additionally, mothers of technology-dependent children report poor physical and mental health, decreased social functioning and increased bodily pain. Approximately half the women studied reported elevated levels of depressive symptoms (Thyen et al., 1998) and very few report practicing wellness habits such as eating balanced diet, exercising regularly and getting sufficient rest (Kuster and Merkle, 2004).

In a longitudinal study of spousal caregiving as a risk factor of mortality, participants who were providing care and experiencing caregiver strain had mortality risks that were 63% higher than non-caregiving controls (Schulz and Beach, 1999). However, those providing care but not reporting strain did not have elevated levels of mortality. These results indicate that there are mediating factors between the caregiving role and poor outcomes. The TSC model may provide us with a framework for understanding the social, cognitive and coping processes that mediate adjustment as an outcome.

Parents of cancer survivors may be particularly at risk for impaired physical and mental health. There is growing evidence that long-term caregivers suffer from decreased overall health. The intense, long-term caregiving relationship elicited by parenting a cancer survivor exceeds that of parenting a healthy child. Indeed, parents of cancer survivors may experience a more intense and prolonged caregiving relationship with their children than parents of other chronically ill children. One study noted that more than 60% of young adult survivors continue to be accompanied to long term follow up visits by parent, more than three times the rate observed for young adults attending a diabetes clinic (Ressler et al., 2003). A more recent study compared parents of adult survivors of pediatric cancer who continued to accompany their children to long-term follow-up clinic appointments and parents of current pediatric cancer patients on or within one year of active treatment (Hardy et al., in press). The parents of adult survivors reported just as much anxiety and illness-related stress as parents of children on active treatment. These results suggest that parents who continue to accompany their young adult child to clinic may remain psychologically vulnerable many years after the end of treatment and that the impact of having a child with a life-threatening illness may not diminish even years into the child's survivorship.

Few studies have specifically focused on health and wellness outcomes in parents of cancer survivors. One study followed parents of childhood cancer patients for a period of 18 months and found no improvement in parent physical and mental well-being over time (Svavarsdottir, 2005). However, one small Taiwanese study compared the physical health of parents of children in active treatment and parents of children off-treatment (Chien et al., 2003). They found that while parents of children of treatment reported better overall health and well-being than parents of children in active treatment, their health was poorer than a normative sample. Clearly, further research on parents of cancer survivors is necessary to better understand the mechanisms through which parents appraise and cope with the strain of parenting a cancer survivor, and how parenting stress in this population may influence their physical and mental health.

Caregiver Stress in a Disability Population

There is much still to be learned about caregiver stress in caregivers of pediatric cancer survivors. This population is incredibly unique. In many ways they are similar to other chronic illness populations. However, for some pediatric cancer survivors, there is less stress related to physical health and illness demands and more stress related to the cognitive late effects and resultant academic and social difficulties associated with these effects. Yet, to date, there have been few interventions aimed at preventing or ameliorating this stress. Therefore, an examination of caregiver stress in a population of parents facing similar stressors, such as parents of children with learning or mild intellectual or development disabilities, may be fruitful in understanding the complex landscape of parenting a pediatric cancer survivor.

Caregiver stress associated with parenting a child with a mental disability, such as a learning disability, intellectual disability, or developmental disability has been studied more extensively to date than survivors of pediatric cancer and their families. Although disabilities may lack some of the emotional salience of the cancer experience, the literature on parent adjustment to parenting a child with a disability may serve to better our understanding of the experience of parenting a survivor of pediatric cancer. Indeed, caregiver stress in this population is qualitatively similar to that associated with raising a childhood cancer survivor. Both populations may experience a sense of loss and grief as they alter their long term hopes and dreams for their child. Similarly, both populations have to deal with an uncertain future for their child that may or may not involve secondary education, a career, or marriage and children. Pragmatically, both populations must advocate for their children in the school system to ensure that they have the best, most appropriate and most comprehensive services available.

Sources of Stress

A study of the experiences of families of children with learning disabilities reveal similar dynamics to those predicted to occur in families of cancer survivors (Dyson, 1996). Specific struggles reported include parents spending an excessive amount of time and energy on the child with a learning disability, sometimes at the cost of spending less time with the non-learning disabled child. Additionally, some parents, particularly high professionally achieving parents, struggle to accept their child's disability and cognitive limitations. Similar to cancer survivors, these parents also expressed concern over their child's social functioning. Indeed, the most notable problems reported by parents were the learning and social difficulties experienced by the child.

There is significant stress associated with receiving an accurate diagnosis of "learning disabled," and the subsequent process of attaining the necessary services. Parental dissatisfaction with the initial delay in diagnosis, frustration with the prolonged process of finding appropriate programs for the children and the financial cost of quality assessment and interventions were three of the most frequently described stressors in Dyson's (1996) study. Similarly, parents reported ongoing stress related to concerns about their child's academic experiences, such as negative report cards, absence of appropriate academic materials, inflexible policies, and reduced teacher attention due to workload.

Similar to the cancer survivorship population, there is a significant amount of variability in the psychological adjustment of parents of children with disabilities. As such, the research focus has shifted from a deficit model to a model of resilience and coping in order to better understand why some families display such hardiness in the face of stress. Many models of parenting stress and adjustment in the disability population include similar parent variables, such as cognitions and coping, as the transactional stress and coping model of adjustment to chronic illness proposed by Thompson and Gustafson (1996). In addition, many interventions have been tested to reduce the caregiver stress associated with parenting a child with a disability. Understanding the variables that contribute to caregiver stress in the disability population is essential to designing research to better understand and intervene with parents of cancer survivors.

The majority of the literature on parenting stress in parents of disabled children is based on a model designed by Abidin (1995), and indicates that these parents do indeed experience elevated levels of stress. One study examined the levels of parental stress among mothers of learning disabled, emotionally impaired and regular school children (Fuller and Rankin, 1994). Overall, mothers of learning disabled children had moderately elevated scores on most subscales. Their mean score on the Parenting Stress Index (PSI) was in the 75th percentile, with items related to the Child Domain in the 90th percentile and the Parent Domain in the 55th percentile. A few subscales showed extremely high levels (90-95th percentile) of stress, including: *acceptability, demandingness* and *reinforcement* in the Child Domain, and a*ttachment* in the Parent Domain. Elevations in the Child Domain indicate that parents of learning disabled children perceived their children's behaviors as difficult to cope with. The elevated *acceptability* subscale indicates that these parents do not feel that their children meet their expectations in terms of emotional, physical or intellectual characteristics. They also perceive their children to be more demanding of them than parents of non-learning disabled children. The elevated *reinforcement* subscale indicates that these parents do not perceive their relationship with their learning disabled child as positively as other parents, and that the interaction does not produce good feelings between them. This sentiment is also reflected in the elevated score on the *attachment* subscale, which could indicate a lack of emotional closeness or an inability of the parent to understand and interpret the child's needs. These elevations clearly place parents of learning disabled children at high risk for clinical levels of parenting-related distress and dysfunctional parent-child interactions.

Despite the overall elevated levels of parenting stress, there is significant variability in the adjustment and adaptation in parents of children with disabilities. Indeed, one recent review of parental adjustment to having a child with a developmental disability revealed many families achieve successful, adaptive functioning and believe their lives are enriched by their disabled child (Kwai-sang Yau and Cecilia, 1999). Some families report a greater emphasis on personal growth and more positive and cohesive family relations as a result of coping with their child's learning disability (Dyson, 1996). This appears to be true even in the case of severe disabilities. Indeed, there is empirical evidence that positive adaptation appears unrelated to the severity of the child's disability (Trute, 1995; Trute and Hauch, 1988). This result parallels the chronic illness literature, in which illness severity has not proven to be a significant predictor of parental adaptation (REF). Similar to parents of chronically ill children, the variables with the most consistent evidence for predicting adjustment are the maternal mediational processes, including parent cognitions, coping, social support and family functioning.

Maternal Mediational Characteristics

Much of the variability in parental adjustment can be attributed to the available intrapersonal resources of the parent. Indeed, two recent reviews of the literature on adaptive functioning in parents reveals that having a positive view and realistic expectations of the child with the disability, a feeling of positive reward associated with parenting, less negative ideation, more ability to creatively respond to the challenges of parenting, and better problem solving skills all predict better adjustment (Kwai-sang Yau and Cecilia, 1999; Scorgie, Wilgosh, and McDonald, 1998). Similar to the literature on adaptation to chronic illness, most of the predictive characteristics are related to cognitions, coping and social support.

Cognitions

Parenting stress has been linked to parent psychological distress, including depression. One study of the psychological adaptation of parents of young, developmentally disabled children found that appraisal of the child's disability as a stressor, personal self-esteem and a strong spousal relationship were significant predictors of depression in mothers and fathers (Trute, 1995). Overall, mothers showed more symptoms of depression than fathers, perhaps due to their highly demanding role as primary caregiver in most traditionally structured families. When mothers filled the role of full time homemaker, Trute (1995) found that their level of depression was mediated by their self esteem and personal coping resources.

Self esteem was also found to play a key role in predicting parenting stress in a sample of mothers of children with mild to moderate intellectual disabilities (Hassall, Rose, and McDonald, 2005). Specifically, lower levels of parenting stress correlated with higher levels of parental satisfaction and parental competence. Parent locus of control was also predictive of parenting stress; mothers with more external locus of control displayed higher levels of parenting stress. In this study, it also appeared that locus of control acted as a mediator of family support on parenting stress, indicating that the direct effect of family support may be contributing to a more internal locus of control for mothers of children with intellectual disabilities (Hassall et al., 2005).

Coping

Hastings and colleagues (Hastings, Allen, McDermott, and Still, 2002) examined factors related to positive perceptions in mothers of children with intellectual disabilities. Reframing coping strategies was associated with numerous positive outcomes, including mother's perceptions of the child as a source of happiness, fulfillment, strength and family closeness. Mothers' perceptions of the child as a source of personal growth and maturity were also positively associated with reframing coping strategies, report of helpfulness and usefulness of social support from family and friends, and perceived caregiving demands.

Individual coping styles may impact overall family functioning and marital satisfaction as well. A study of families of young children with a variety of mental disabilities found that emotion-focused coping such as wishful thinking, self-blame, distancing and self-control were negatively related to family strengths (Judge, 1998). Successful use of social support was highly associated with family strengths. A similar study revealed that fathers who employed more problem-focused coping strategies were more positive about their marriages, and that wives also reported higher marital adjustment when their husbands employed problem focused strategies (Stoneman and Gavidia-Payne, 2006). Overall, these results support a relationship between problem-focused coping and parental positive perceptions that may be clinically important for supporting families under similar stress.

Social Support

Environmental characteristics such as family socio-economic status, social support and family functioning have been linked to parent adjustment (Kwai-sang Yau and Cecilia, 1999; Scorgie et al., 1998; Trute, 1995). Unsurprisingly, families in higher socio-economic status groups tend to have more financial stability to cope with the extra health and daily living demands associated with raising a child with a disability, and a higher level of educational achievement. A supportive social network and positive family functioning also contribute to parent adjustment and adaptation. Similarly, two parent households with fewer children also have more resources available (Kwai-sang Yau and Cecilia, 1999).

Social support has consistently been linked to positive adaptation and lower levels of parenting stress in families of children with disabilities (Hassall et al., 2005). A review of parent adjustment indicates that it is the parent's satisfaction with their perceived support rather than the amount of support per se that is an important predictor of adjustment (Kwai-sang Yau and Cecilia, 1999). Indeed a small group of very supportive individuals may be adequate for some parents as a study of parents with young, developmentally disabled children found (Trute, 1995). The families in this study tended to have fairly sparse social networks with very focused involvement from a few close friends and family members (Trute, 1995). Parental skill in utilizing networks of extended family, friends and professional resources also appears to be highly relevant to successful adaptation. In fact, a parent's ability to access and coordinate a small network of intense connections in response to stress or crisis has been linked to successful adaptation to the birth of a developmentally disabled child (Trute and Hauch, 1988). This study also maintained that supportive relationships in families of disabled children tend to be multidimensional. That is, contacts can serve multiple functions such as sharing in social activities, providing practical help like respite care, and financial aid (Trute and Hauch, 1988).

Social support also appears to be connected to family functioning. Parent satisfaction with support and the number of sources of support were shown to be positively related to family integrity, lowered stress, parent perceptions of child functioning, parent-child interaction and child behavior (Kwai-sang Yau and Cecilia, 1999). In a study of families that positively adapted to the birth of a developmentally disabled child, Trute and Hauch (1988) found that these families had unusually well established support systems in both the social and family domain. In two-parent households in particular, there was a high level of cohesion, in that both parents maintained mutual contacts and shared relationships with others.

One study examined family functioning as measured by caregiver expressed emotion, appraisal of behavior problems, and parenting stress in a sample of caregivers of school-aged children with learning disabilities (Lam, Giles, and Lavander, 2003). Expressed emotion was found to mediate the relationship between the child's disability and caregiver stress. Specifically, high expressed emotion caregivers appraised more of their children's behavior as "problematic", and perceived their social support to be less adequate. In contrast, high warmth was related to more positive reappraisal and less-escape avoidance, two coping strategies typically associated with positive adaptation. Mother's appraisal of their child's disability and behavior as a stressor plays a significant role in the coping process.

Clearly, there is strong evidence to suggest similar mediational processes in the adjustment to parenting a child with learning disabilities and the adjustment to parenting a pediatric cancer survivor. In both situations, maternal cognitions, particularly those involved in appraisal of the situation as a stressor, coping style, and availability of appropriate social support all predict maternal adjustment. Now that we have reviewed the evidence for the similarity between the two populations, we will now examine interventions used in the disability population that could serve as models for designing interventions in the cancer survivor population.

Interventions

Although problems related to pediatric cancer survivorship are relatively new, problems related to learning disabilities have been well studied. Indeed, many interventions both with children with disabilities and their parents have been implemented with much success. These interventions have already begun to inform treatment of pediatric cancer survivors. It is time now to consider how stress reduction interventions for parents of children with learning disabilities may serve to enlighten our treatment of parents of pediatric cancer survivors.

One of the first areas in which psycho-oncology leveraged the extensive body of knowledge we have about children with learning disabilities is in the treatment of attentional deficits. The attentional deficits exhibited by pediatric cancer survivors are indeed similar to those of children diagnosed with Attention Deficit/Hyperactivity Disorder (ADHD). ADHD is a serious disorder that affects approximately 4-6% of the child population (APA, 1994). It is associated with many short- and long-term impairments, such as impulsivity and difficulty concentrating, which may contribute to increased stress related to the parenting role. In recent years, interventions for children with ADHD have begun to inform the conceptualization and treatment of survivors of pediatric cancer with neurocognitive impairments.

Children with ADHD (who are otherwise healthy) have been treated effectively over the past 50 years with stimulant medication, such as methylphenidate hydrochloride (MPH; popularly known as Ritalin), to improve their cognitive performance (Brown, Dingle, and Dreelin, 1997; Hechtman et al., 2004; Klein, Abikoff, Hechtman, and Weiss, 2004). Specifically, MPH has improved performance on measures of vigilance and sustained attention, reaction time, paired association learning and perceptual efficiency. MPH has also been shown to improve social skills, as rated by peer ratings and behavioral observation, in children with ADHD (Brown et al., 1997). Two recent randomized trials have examined the efficacy of MPH in a specific subset of childhood cancer survivors that display academic achievement problems and attention problems (Conklin et al., in press; Mulhern et al., 2004; S. Thompson, Leigh, and Christensen, 2001).

Thompson and colleagues (2001) were the first to study the effects of MPH on pediatric cancer survivors in a small (n = 32) randomized, double blind trial. The group receiving MPH displayed significantly greater improvement on a computerized continuous performance test of attentional functioning. Mulhern et al. (2004) extended this work to larger sample (n = 83) of long-term cancer survivors identified as having attentional deficits and problems with academic achievement. This study was also randomized and double blind, but included groups of placebo, low-dose MPH and moderate-dose MPH. The two MPH groups did not differ significantly from each other. However, significant improvement with MPH was reported by teachers and parents on measures of attentional and social functioning. Conklin and colleagues (in press) replicated these findings in a larger (n=122), two-day, in clinic, double blind, crossover trial in which survivors of childhood cancer with learning impairments received either MPH or a placebo. A significant MPH vs. placebo effect was revealed on a measure of attention, cognitive flexibility and processing speed. No adverse side effects were reported. These results indicate that some survivors of pediatric cancer may benefit from low doses of MPH, and provide further evidence for the similarity in the cognitive and social functioning of children with ADHD and childhood cancer survivors.

Similarly, educational services for pediatric cancer survivors often resemble those implemented for children with learning disabilities. Butler and Copeland (2002) have developed a three part model, the Cognitive Remediation Program (CRP) to address neurocognitive deficits in pediatric cancer survivors that draws on three disciplines: special education/educational psychology, brain injury rehabilitation and clinical psychology. The educational components of CRP involve instruction on fifteen different metacognitive strategies in the areas of task preparedness, on-task performance and post-task strategies. From the brain injury rehabilitation domain, this intervention uses massed practice to exercise and retrain attentional processes. From the clinical psychology domain, this intervention takes a cognitive behavioral approach, and leverages strategies such as reframing struggles into a positive light and monitoring internal dialogue. These methods are specifically targeted at improving the ability to withstand distraction. Pilot data from this intervention suggests that this team-based, multi-dimensional approach is effective in reducing attentional deficits in pediatric cancer survivors.

Both the methylphenidate and cognitive rehabilitation interventions are examples of researchers borrowing from the extensive body of research on children with learning disabilities to treat children who have survived cancer. Given the similar sources of stress and mediational variables predicting parental outcome, it would be useful to examine interventions aimed at reducing parenting stress in the disability population to inform our work with parents of cancer survivors. To date, most interventions aimed at stress reduction for parents of children with disabilities have targeted parents' intrapersonal resources through cognitive behavioral approaches. In addition, many have been group-based interventions, the design of which inherently addresses social support deficits.

Parents in both groups share comparable challenges in receiving appropriate support. One of the most socially significant and challenging aspects of a learning disability is that it may be hidden and seemingly benign (Dyson, 1993). Similarly, little is known in the general population regarding potential cognitive late effects of cancer. This potential invisibility of this disability can lead to delayed or conflicting diagnoses, which interferes with intervention and ability to engage appropriate services (Dyson, 1996). In parents, it can also lead to confusion, ambivalence or unrealistic expectations for the child's academic success (Dyson, 1996). One place that parents can turn is to other parents who are dealing with a similar situation. Indeed, participation in parent support groups has been linked to adjustment and adaptation of parents of children with learning and intellectual disabilities (Kwai-sang Yau and Cecilia, 1999).

Parent support groups may be similarly useful for parents of cancer survivors. Indeed, Kazak and colleagues (2004) recently successfully implemented a one day cognitive-behavioral family based group intervention aimed at reducing posttraumatic stress symptoms in survivors and their families. Similar group based interventions aimed at reducing overall caregiving stress may be particularly helpful to this population, whose concerns about academic performance in survivors may seem secondary, or even "invisible," to others, whose focus may be on the child's survival or medical outcomes. It may not occur to those unfamiliar with cancer that late effects do impact child academic and social functioning, and that they may result in ongoing grief, loss or stress for parents long after the disease has been "cured." Parent support groups promote understanding and offer parents therapeutic involvement with people who are experiencing similar situations. In groups, parents can discuss their concerns and exchange ideas with each other thereby facilitating parents acting as advocates on their own behalf and the behalf of their child with special needs (Kwai-sang Yau and Cecilia, 1999). Ideally, with this support, parents will start to act as decision makers and as independent policy planners. The emergence of parents as involved, outspoken advocates has the potential to have considerable impact on service provision for special need children in the educational system.

A recent review of stress reduction interventions for parents of children with intellectual disabilities suggests that the strongest evidence is for cognitive behavioral group interventions in reducing parenting stress and improving mental health (Hastings and Beck, 2004). Although the six interventions the article reviewed were varied, they all utilized a group format and cognitive behavioral techniques, including problem-solving, cognitive restructuring, and monitoring thoughts and feelings. Some also included non-cognitive behavioral techniques, including educational/information provision, relaxation, and systemic family therapy.

An example of a successful, multi-component intervention is the "Caring for Parent Caregiver" program, a family-focused intervention designed to empower the individual and thereby strengthen family resources (Schultz, Kemm, Bruce, and Smyrnios, 1992; Schultz, Schultz, Bruce, Smyrnios, and et al., 1993). This intervention, comprised of six weekly 2-hour sessions, aimed to provide a model for expression of feelings, increased awareness of personal strengths, development of strategies and skills in problem-solving, and enlargement of external sources for support. Immediately post-treatment, a qualitative analysis of participant response was completed. Participants reported enhanced personal skills, as well as changes in insight and interpersonal relationships. Attitudinal changes included improved self-esteem, self-confidence and a more positive approach to challenges. Behavioral changes included increased communication, coping, stress-management skills, and improved problem-solving abilities (Schultz et al., 1992). Twelve months post-treatment, program participants displayed less emotional distress than control group subjects, and continued to report very high overall satisfaction with the program (Schultz et al., 1993).

One recent study examined the effectiveness of counseling groups in reducing stress of parents with learning disabilities (Shechtman and Gilat, 2005). The counseling group was compared to an educational group that focused on attitudes, levels of stress and sense of control. The counseling group consisted of twelve 90-minute sessions. The initial three sessions were structured around the goals of establishing group norms, rapport and cohesiveness. The middle six sessions was the "working stage" in which members shared their unique difficulties related to their child with a learning disability. These sessions typically resulted in high levels of self disclosure and emotional experiencing. The final stage (3 sessions) was focused on helping mothers cope with the difficulties through guidance and information provision. In contrast, the education-didactic group, which was considered the standard of care intervention, consisted of eight 90-minute sessions in which the goal was to provide information on learning disabilities as a means of facilitating better coping. The sessions were typically a lecture format with time for questions. Overall, results indicated greater gains over time for patients in the counseling group on measures of parenting stress, parenting attitudes, and parenting locus of control. These results indicate that provision of information alone is an insufficient intervention for this population, and that the unique therapeutic effects of group counseling may better meet these parents' needs.

A few tentative conclusions may be drawn from the results of these intervention studies. Implementing a structured intervention to target parenting stress appears to have a positive impact over standard services. A group format provides parents opportunities to serve as a support system for other parents in similar circumstances, which can be effective in reducing parenting stress. In particular, group interventions that incorporate cognitive behavioral techniques are especially effective at reducing parental stress and improving mental health. Considering the similar sources of stress in parents of learning disabled children and parents of cancer survivors, future research on parents of survivors may be informed by these conclusions. We have preliminary evidence that parents of cancer survivors experience elevated levels of psychological distress and parenting-related stress on an ongoing basis. A recent meta-analysis of pediatric cancer interventions found significant effects in interventions aimed at decreasing distress and improving the adjustment of parents of children with cancer at all stages of treatment (Pai, Drotar, Zebracki, Moore, and Youngstrom, 2006). These promising results indicate that parents of cancer survivors would likely benefit from interventions targeted at reducing distress and improving adjustment. Future research should continue to examine the mediational processes that impact parental adjustment to survivorship. If the hypothesized cognitive, coping and social support mediators are found to apply to this population, inventions may then be designed, in part informed by the disability interventions, to potentially ameliorate the stress of this unique population.

Conclusion

Parenting involves a dynamic balance of resources and demands. While some degree of stress associated with the parenting role is inevitable, some parents face additional stressors that challenge their flexibility and resourcefulness. Parents of pediatric cancer survivors are one subgroup of parents that deal with chronic stressors related to their role as caregiver. Indeed, these parents must provide emotional support to their children, while simultaneously processing their own fears and emotions. These parents must also face the uncertainty of newly emerging neurocognitive late effects as a result of their child's treatment. When neurocognitive deficits do emerge, these parents are called upon to act as advocates for their children to ensure they are receiving adequate assessment and intervention in the educational system. Interestingly, there is significant variability in the psychological adjustment in this group of parents that is not directly related to their child's disease severity. While some parents are able to report a greater sense of meaning and personal growth as a result of the cancer experience, others struggle with ongoing grief and uncertainty. Although most survivors and their families adjust relatively well, there may be subtle long term effects of chronic stress that are not sensitively measured by clinical assessment tools.

The transactional stress and coping model, proposed by Thompson and Gustafson (1996) to describe maternal adjustment in mothers of children with chronic illness, provides a framework within which this variability can be understood. They propose several maternal mediational variables that have been empirically validated to predict maternal adjustment, including maternal cognitions, coping style and family functioning. There is also evidence within the disability literature to support these variables as mediators of the parental stress and coping processes. Indeed, this dual support from the chronic illness and disability fields are quite compelling for the survivor population. Pediatric cancer survivorship currently falls at the crossroads of chronic illness and learning disability, particularly for those children treated with intrathecal methotrexate or cranial radiation.

There has been a call for evidence-based interventions during and after treatment that address cancer-specific psychosocial sequelae (Kazak, 2005). Interventions targeting parenting stress would be well served by learning from the success of group-based cognitive behavioral interventions aimed at reducing stress in parents of children with disabilities. In doing so, interventions for parents should be group-based to enhance the sense of community amongst these parents. Group dynamics enable mobilization of advocacy actions, as well as provide social support. Interventions should specifically target salient attributes known to mediate the stress process, including parent cognitions like locus of control, child attributions and self-efficacy. This may be achieved through psycho-education about late effects, child development, learning disabilities, and educational services, which would increase knowledge and provide more realistic expectations for child behavior. In addition, adaptive or active coping techniques should be taught. In particular, problem-solving and reframing techniques should be emphasized to encourage a sense of personal strength and growth.

As the numbers of pediatric cancer survivors continue to increase, the need for psychosocial research on adjustment and its predictors becomes increasingly relevant. While a thorough examination of parenting stress in parents of long-term pediatric cancer survivors is called for to better understand and treat these families, we can say with confidence that this group of parents faces significant ongoing stress. Currently, little is being done to assist these parents in coping with the unique set of stressors associated with cancer experience. Targeting those variables that are known to predict positive adaptation to the stress of parenting a cancer survivor will serve to benefit caregivers and survivors alike. While parenting stress is clearly detrimental for caregivers, it also impacts the survivors themselves. Parents of survivors continue to maintain an active parenting role even as survivors enter young adulthood, and their behavior will have an ongoing influence over their children's development. In addition, caregivers serve as proxies of their children's behalves in much psychosocial research, and their stress may be reflected in their responses.

Interventions aimed at parents of cancer survivors must respect that each individual and family is unique with their own set of needs and concerns, as these families are not a homogenous group. Indeed, the existing research on parents of children with mental disabilities and parents of cancer survivors share in the complexity of working with very heterogeneous samples. Similarly, for any given parent, adaptation is not necessarily a linear process. Learning to appreciate a child's unique abilities does not mean that parents will no longer have intense and conflicting feelings related to having a child with a disability. Indeed, critical events and times of transition in the family life cycle, such as beginning or changing schools, may result in the re-emergence of feelings. Interventions should have two main objectives: 1) to enhance a sense of community and empower the community to act as advocates; and 2) to strengthen parent attributes and characteristics that promote successful coping and adaptation. Pediatric cancer is a stressful experience for any parent to face. However, this stress does not end with the eradication of the cancer and the completion of treatment. As such, the increasing number of survivors provides an opportunity to develop and implement interventions to provide families with a sense of hope and meaning from an otherwise difficult experience.

References

Abidin, R. R. (1995). *Parenting Stress Index (PSI) manual (3rd Edition)*. Lutz, FL: Psychological Assessment Resources, Inc.

Alderfer, M. A., Cnaan, A., Annunziato, R. A., and Kazak, A. E. (2005). Patterns of Posttraumatic Stress Symptoms in Parents of Childhood Cancer Survivors. *Journal of Family Psychology, 19*(3), 430-440.

American Cancer Society. (2007). *Cancer Facts and Figures*. Atlanta, GA.

APA. (1994). *Diagnostic and Statistical Manual of the American Psychiatric Association*: American Psychiatric Association.

Armstrong, F., and Mulhern, R. K. (1999). Acute Lymphoblastic Leukemia and Brain Tumors. In R. T. Brown (Ed.), *Cognitive aspects of chronic illness in children*. New York, NY: The Guilford Press.

Baker, D. B., and McCal, K. (1995). Parenting stress in parents of children with attention-deficit hyperactivity disorder and parents of children with learning disabilities. *Journal of Child and Family Studies, 4*(1), 57-68.

Bandura, A. (1977). Self-efficacy: Toward a unifying theory of behavioral change. *Psychological Review, 84*, 191-215.

Bonner, M. J., Hardy, K. K., Guill, A. B., McLaughlin, C., Schweitzer, H., and Carter, K. (2006). Development and validation of the parent experience of child illness. *Journal of Pediatric Psychology, 31*(3), 310-321.

Bonner, M. J., Hardy, K. K., Willard, V. W., and Hutchinson, K. C. (2007). Brief report: psychosocial functioning of fathers as primary caregivers of pediatric oncology patients. *Journal of Pediatric Psychology, 32*(7), 851-856.

Bonner, M. J., Hardy, K. K., Willard, V. W., Hutchinson, K. C., and Guill, A. B. (in press). Further validation of the Parent Experience of Child Illness (PECI) Scale. *Children's Health Care.*

Bronfenbrenner, U. (1986). Ecology of the family as a context for human development: Research perspectives. *Developmental Psychology, 22*(6), 723-742.

Brown, R. T., Daly, B. P., and Rickel, A. U. (2007). *Chronic Illness in Children and Adolescents.* Cambridge, MA: Hogrefe and Huber Publishers.

Brown, R. T., Dingle, A., and Dreelin, B. (1997). Neuropsychological effects of stimulant medication on children's learning behavior. In C. Reynolds and E. Fletcher-Janzen (Eds.), *Handbook of clinical child pharmacology.* New York, NY: Wiley.

Brown, R. T., Madan-Swain, A., and Lambert, R. (2003). Posttraumatic stress symptoms in adolescent survivors of childhood cancer and their mothers. *Journal of Traumatic Stress, 16*(4), 309-318.

Brown, R. T., Madan-Swain, A., R, P., Lambert, R., Sexson, S., and Ragab, A. (1992). Chemotherapy for acute lymphocytic leukemia: Cognitive and academic sequelae. *Journal of Pediatric Psychology, 121*, 885-889.

Buono, L. A., Morris, M. K., Morris, R. D., Krawiecki, N., Norris, F. H., Foster, M. A., et al. (1998). Evidence for the Syndrome of Nonverbal Learning Disabilities in Children with Brain Tumors. *Child Neuropsychology, 4*, 144-157.

Burke, M., Hainsworth, M., Eakes, G., and Lindgren, C. (1992). Current knowledge and research on chronic sorrow: A foundation for inquiry. *Death Studies, 16*(231-245).

Butler, R. W., and Copeland, D. R. (2002). Attentional processes and their remediation in children treated for cancer: a literature review and the development of a therapeutic approach. *Journal of the International Neuropsychological Society, 8*(1), 115-124.

Butler, R. W., and Mulhern, R. K. (2005). Neurocognitive interventions for children and adolescents surviving cancer. *Journal of Pediatric Psychology, 30*(1), 65-78.

Carey, M. E., Barakat, L. P., Foley, B., Gyato, K., and Phillips, P. C. (2001). Neuropsychological functioning and social functioning of survivors of pediatric brain tumors: evidence of nonverbal learning disability. *Child Neuropsychology, 7*(4), 265-272.

Chien, L.-Y., Lo, L.-H., Chen, C.-J., Chen, Y.-C., Chiang, C.-C., and Yu Chao, Y.-M. (2003). Quality of life among primary caregivers of Taiwanese children with brain tumor. *Cancer Nursing, 26*(4), 305-311.

Cohen, M. H. (1995). The triggers of heightened parental uncertainty in chronic, life-threatening childhood illness. *Qualitative Health Research Vol. 5(1) Feb 1995, 63-77.*

Cohen, S., Doyle, W. J., and Skoner, D. P. (1999). Psychological stress, cytokine production, and severity of upper respiratory illness. *Psychosomatic Medicine, 61*(2), 175-180.

Cohen, S., Tyrrell, D. A., and Smith, A. P. (1991). Psychological stress and susceptibility to the common cold. *New England Journal of Medicine, 325*(9), 606-612.

Cohen, S., and Williamson, G. M. (1991). Stress and infectious disease in humans. *Psychological Bulletin, 109*(1), 5-24.

Conklin, H. M., Khan, R. B., Reddick, W. E., Helton, S., Brown, R. T., Howard, S. C., et al. (in press). Acute Neurocognitive Response to Methylphenidate Among Survivors of

Childhood Cancer: A Randomized, Double-Blind, Cross-Over Trial. *Journal of Pediatric Psychology.*

Copeland, D. R., Moore, B. D., Francis, D., Jaffe, N., and Culbert, S. (1996). Neuropsychological effects of chemotherapy on children with cancer: A longitudinal study. *Journal of Clinical Oncology, 14*, 2826-2835.

Crnic, K. A., and Greenberg, M. T. (1990). Minor parenting stresses with young children. *Child Development, 61*(5), 1628-1637.

Dennis, M., Speigler, B. L., Hoffman, J. J., Hendrick, E. B., Humphreys, R. P., and Chaung, S. (1991). Brain tumors in children and adolescents: the neuroanatomy of deficits in working, associative and serial order memory. *Neuropsychologia, 29*, 829-847.

Dix, T. (1993). Attributing dispositions to children: An interactional analysis of attribution in socialization. *Personality and Social Psychology Bulletin Vol. 19(5) Oct 1993, 633-643.*

Dix, T., Ruble, D. N., Grusec, J. E., and Nixon, S. (1986). Social cognition in parents: Inferential and affective reactions to children of three age levels. *Child Development, 57*(4), 879-894.

Dyson, L. L. (1993). Response to the presence of a child with disabilities: parental stress and family functioning over time. *American Journal of Mental Retardation, 98*(2), 207-218.

Dyson, L. L. (1996). The experiences of families of children with learning disabilities: Parental stress, family functioning, and sibling self-concept. *Journal of Learning Disabilities Vol 29(3) May 1996, 280-286.*

Eiser, C. (1998). Practitioner review: Long-term consequences of childhood cancer. *Journal of Child Psychology and Psychiatry, 39*(5), 621-633.

Finney, J. W., and Bonner, M. J. (1992). The influence of behavioral family intervention on children's health and health care use. *Behavioral Change, 9*, 157-170.

Folkman, S., and Lazarus, R. S. (1988). Coping as a mediator of emotion. *Journal of Personality and Social Psychology, 54*(3), 466-475.

Folkman, S., Lazarus, R. S., Gruen, R., and DeLongis, A. (1986). Appraisal, coping, health status and psychological symptoms. *Journal of Personality and Social Psychology, 50*(3), 571-579.

Frank, N. C., Brown, R. T., Blount, R. L., and Bunke, V. (2001). Predictors of affective responses of mothers and fathers of children with cancer. *Psycho-Oncology, 10*(4), 293-304.

Fuller, G. B., and Rankin, R. E. (1994). Differences in levels of parental stress among mothers of learning disabled, emotionally impaired, and regular school children. *Perceptual and Motor Skills Vol 78(2) Apr 1994, 583-592.*

Goldbeck, L. (2001). Parental coping with the diagnosis of childhood cancer: Gender effects, dissimilarity within couples, and quality of life. *Psycho-Oncology, 10*, 325-335.

Goldberg, S., Morris, P., Simmons, R. J., Fowler, R. S., and et al. (1990). Chronic illness in infancy and parenting stress: A comparison of three groups of parents. *Journal of Pediatric Psychology, 15*(3), 347-358.

Hardy, K. K., Bonner, M. J., Masi, R., Hutchinson, K. C., Willard, V. W., and Rosoff, P. M. (in press). Psychosocial functioning in parents of adult survivors of childhood cancer. *Journal of Pediatric Hematology and Oncology.*

Hassall, R., Rose, J., and McDonald, J. (2005). Parenting stress in mothers of children with an intellectual disability: The effects of parental cognitions in relation to child characteristics and family support. *Journal of Intellectual Disability Research, 49*(6), 405-418.

Hastings, R. P., Allen, R., McDermott, K., and Still, D. (2002). Factors related to positive perceptions in mothers of children with intellectual disabilities. *Journal of Applied Research in Intellectual Disabilities Vol. 15(3) 2002, 269-275.*

Hastings, R. P., and Beck, A. (2004). Practitioner Review: Stress intervention for parents of children with intellectual disabilities. *Journal of Child Psychology and Psychiatry, 45*(8), 1338-1349.

Hechtman, L., Abikoff, H., Klein, R. G., Greenfield, B., Etcovitch, J., Cousins, L., et al. (2004). Children with ADHD treated with long-term methylphenidate and multimodal psychosocial treatment: Impact on parental practices. *Journal of the American Academy of Child and Adolescent Psychiatry, 43*(7), 830-838.

Herbert, T. B., and Cohen, S. (1993). Stress and immunity in humans: a meta-analytic review. *Psychosomatic Medicine, 55*(4), 364-379.

Hill, J., Kondryn, H., Mackie, E., McNally, R., and Eden, T. (2003). Adult psychosocial functioning following childhood cancer: the different roles of sons' and daughters' relationships with their fathers and mothers. *Journal of Child Psychology and Psychiatry, 44*(5), 752-762.

Horwitz, W., and Kazak, A. E. (1990). Family adaptation to childhood cancer: Sibling and family systems variables. *Journal of Clinical Child Psychology, 19*, 221-228.

Houtzager, B., Oort, F., Hoekstra-Weebers, J. E., Caron, H., Grootenhuis, M., and Last, B. (2004). Coping and family functioning predict longitudinal psychological adaptation of siblings of childhood cancer patients. *Journal of Pediatric Psychology, 29*(8), 591-605.

Judge, S. (1998). Parental coping strategies and strengths in families of young children with disabilities. *Family Relations, 47*(3), 263-268.

Kazak, A. E. (1989). Families of chronically ill children: a systems and social-ecological model of adaptation and challenge. *Journal of Consulting and Clinical Psychology, 57*(1), 25-30.

Kazak, A. E. (2005). Evidence-Based Interventions for Survivors of Childhood Cancer and Their Families. *Journal of Pediatric Psychology, 30*(1), 29-39.

Kazak, A. E., Alderfer, M., Rourke, M. T., Simms, S., Streisand, R., and Grossman, J. R. (2004). Posttraumatic stress disorder (PTSD) and posttraumatic stress symptoms (PTSS) in families of adolescent childhood cancer survivors. *Journal of Pediatric Psychology, 29*(3), 211-219.

Kazak, A. E., Alderfer, M. A., Streisand, R., Simms, S., Rourke, M. T., Barakat, L. P., et al. (2004). Treatment of Posttraumatic Stress Symptoms in Adolescent Survivors of Childhood Cancer and Their Families: A Randomized Clinical Trial. *Journal of Family Psychology, 18*(3), 493-504.

Kazak, A. E., and Barakat, L. P. (1997). Brief report: Parenting stress and quality of life during treatment for childhood leukemia predicts child and parent adjustment after treatment ends. *Journal of Pediatric Psychology, 22*(5), 749-758.

Kazak, A. E., Barakat, L. P., Meeske, K., Christakis, D., Meadows, A. T., Casey, R., et al. (1997). Posttraumatic stress, family functioning, and social support in survivors of childhood leukemia and their mothers and fathers. *Journal of Consulting and Clinical Psychology, 65*(1), 120-129.

Kiecolt-Glaser, J. K., Glaser, R., Shuttleworth, E. C., Dyer, C. S., Ogrocki, P., and Speicher, C. E. (1987). Chronic stress and immunity in family caregivers of Alzheimer's disease victims. *Psychosomatic Medicine, 49*(5), 523-535.

Klein, R. G., Abikoff, H., Hechtman, L., and Weiss, G. (2004). Design and rationale of controlled study of long-term methylphenidate and multimodal psychosocial treatment in children with ADHD. *Journal of the American Academy of Child and Adolescent Psychiatry, 43*(7), 792-801.

Kronenberger, W. G., and Thompson, R. J., Jr. (1990). Dimensions of family functioning in families with chronically ill children: A higher order factor analysis of the Family Environment Scale. *Journal of Clinical Child Psychology, 19*(4), 380-388.

Kronenberger, W. G., and Thompson, R. J., Jr. (1992). Psychological adaptation of mothers of children with spina bifida: Association with dimensions of social relationships. *Journal of Pediatric Psychology, 17*(1), 1-14.

Kuster, P. A., Badr, L. K., Chang, B. L., Wuerker, A. K., and Benjamin, A. E. (2004). Factors influencing health promoting activities of mothers caring for ventilator-assisted children. *Journal of Pediatric Nursing, 19*(4), 276-287.

Kuster, P. A., and Merkle, C. J. (2004). Caregiving stress, immune function, and health: Implications for research with parents of medically fragile children. *Issues in Comprehensive Pediatric Nursing, 27*(4), 257-276.

Kwai-sang Yau, M., and Cecilia, W. (1999). Adjustment and adaptation in parents of children with developmental disability in two-parent families: A review of the characteristics and attributes. *British Journal of Developmental Disabilities, 45(88*, 38-51.

Lam, D., Giles, A., and Lavander, A. (2003). Carers' expressed emotion, appraisal of behavioural problems and stress in children attending schools for learning disabilities. *Journal of Intellectual Disability Research, 47*(6), 456-463.

Lazarus, R. S., and Folkman, S. (1984). *Stress, Appraisal, and Coping*. New York, NY: Springer.

Lederber, M. (1998). The family of the cancer patient. In J. Holland (Ed.), *Psycho-Oncology* (pp. 981-1032). New York, NY: Oxford University Press.

Lu, Y. Y.-F., and Austrom, M. G. (2005). Distress Responses and Self-Care Behaviors in Dementia Family Caregivers With High and Low Depressed Mood. *Journal of the American Psychiatric Nurses Association Vol 11(4) Aug 2005, 231-240.*

Madan-Swain, A., Brown, R. T., Foster, M. A., Vega, R., Byars, K., Rodenberger, W., et al. (2000). Identity in adolescent survivors of childhood cancer. *Journal of Pediatric Psychology, 25*(2), 105-115.

McCubbin, M., Balling, K., Possin, P., Frierdich, S., and Bryne, B. (2002). Family resiliency in childhood cancer. *Family Relations, 51*(2), 103-111.

Miller, S. A. (1988). Parents' beliefs about children's cognitive development. *Child Development, 59*, 259-285.

Mishel, M. H. (1981). The measurement of uncertainty in illness. *Nursing Research Vol 30(5) Sep-Oct 1981, 258-263.*

Mishel, M. H. (1983). Parents' perception of uncertainty concerning their hospitalized child. *Nursing Research Vol 32(6) Nov-Dec 1983, 324-330.*

Mishel, M. H. (1988). Uncertainty in illness. *IMAGE: Journal of Nursing Scholarship Vol. 20(4) Win 1988, 225-232.*

Moore, B. D. (2005). Neurocognitive outcomes in survivors of childhood cancer. *Journal of Pediatric Psychology, 30*(1), 51-63.

Moos, R. H., and Tsu, V. D. (1977). The crisis of physical illness: An overview. In R. H. Moos (Ed.), *Coping with physical illness.* (pp. 3-12). New York, NY: Plenum Press.

Mulhern, R. K., Khan, R. B., Kaplan, S., Helton, S., Christensen, R., Bonner, M. J., et al. (2004). Short-term efficacy of methylphenidate: a randomized, double-blind, placebo-controlled trial among survivors of childhood cancer. *Journal of Clinical Oncology, 22*(23), 4795-4803.

Mulhern, R. K., Kovnar, E. H., Kun, L. A., Crisco, J. J., and Williams, J. M. (1988). Phsyiologic and neurologic function following treatment for childhood temporal lobe astrocytoma. *Journal of Child Neurology, 3*, 47-52.

Nagarajan, R., Neglia, J. P., Clohisy, D. R., Yasui, Y., Greenberg, M., Hudson, M., et al. (2003). Education, employment, insurance, and marital status among 694 survivors of pediatric lower extremity bone tumors: a report from the childhood cancer survivor study. *Cancer, 97*(10), 2554-2564.

Naliboff, B. D., Benton, D., Solomon, G. F., Morley, J. E., Fahey, J. L., Bloom, E. T., et al. (1991). Immunological changes in young and old adults during brief laboratory stress. *Psychosomatic Medicine, 53*(2), 121-132.

Norberg, A., Lindbad, F., and Boman, K. (2006). Support-seeking, perceived social support and anxiety in mothers and fathers after children's cancer treatment. *Psycho-oncology, 15*(4), 335-343.

Oeffinger, K. C., and Hudson, M. M. (2004). Long-term complications following childhood and adolescent cancer: foundations for providing risk-based health care for survivors. *CA: a Cancer Journal for Clinicians, 54*(4), 208-236.

Oeffinger, K. C., Mertens, A. C., Hudson, M. M., Gurney, J. G., Casillas, J., Chen, H., et al. (2004). Health care of young adult survivors of childhood cancer: a report from the Childhood Cancer Survivor Study. *Annals of Family Medicine, 2*(1), 61-70.

Pai, A. L. H., Drotar, D., Zebracki, K., Moore, M., and Youngstrom, E. (2006). A meta-analysis of the effects of psychological interventions in pediatric oncology on outcomes of psychological distress and adjustment. *Journal of Pediatric Psychology, 31*(9), 978-988.

Parry, C. (2003). Embracing uncertainty: An exploration of the experiences of childhood cancer survivors. *Qualitative Health Research. 13*(1), 227-246.

Patenaude, A. F., and Kupst, M. J. (2005). Psychosocial Functioning in Pediatric Cancer *Journal of Pediatric Psychology, 30*, 9-27.

Patterson, G. R. (1983). Stress: A change agent for family process. In N. Garmezy and M. Rutter (Eds.), *Stress, coping and development in children.* New York, NY: McGraw Hill.

Patterson, J., Holm, K., and Gurney, J. G. (2004). The impact of childhood cancer on the family: A qualitative analysis of strains, resources and coping behaviors. *Psycho-Oncology, 13*, 390-407.

Peterson, C. C., and Drotar, D. (2006). Family Impact of Neurodevelopmental Late Effects in Survivors of Pediatric Cancer: Review of research, clinical evidence, and future directions. *Clinical Child Psychology and Psychiatry, 11*(3), 349-366.

Pless, P. I., and Pinkerton, P. (1975). *Chronic childhood disorders: Promoting patterns of adjustment.* Chicago, IL: Year-Book Medical Publishers.

Rait, D., Ostroff, J., Smith, K., and Cella, D. (1992). Lives in the balance: Perceived family functioning and the psychosocial adjustment of adolescent cancer survivors. *Family Process, 31*, 383-397.

Ressler, I. B., Cash, J., McNeill, D., Joy, S., and Rosoff, P. M. (2003). Continued parental attendance at a clinic for adult survivors of childhood cancer. *Journal of Pediatric Hematology/Oncology, 25*(11), 868-873.

Robinson, K. E., Gerhardt, C. A., Vannatta, K., and Noll, R. B. (2007). Parent and family factors associated with child adjustment to pediatric cancer. *Journal of Pediatric Psychology, 32*(4), 400-410.

Rubin, K. H., Mills, R. S. L., and Rose-Krasnor, L. (1989). Maternal beliefs and children's social competence. In B. H. Schneider, G. Attili, J. Nadel and R. P. Weissberg (Eds.), *Social competence in developmental perspective.* Dordrecht, The Netherlands: Kluwer Academic.

Sahler, O. J. Z., Fairclough, D. L., Phipps, S., Mulhern, R. K., Dolgin, M. J., Noll, R. B., et al. (2005). Using Problem-Solving Skills Training to Reduce Negative Affectivity in Mothers of Children With Newly Diagnosed Cancer: Report of a Multisite Randomized Trial. *Journal of Consulting and Clinical Psychology, 73*(2), 272-283.

Sahler, O. J. Z., Varni, J. W., Fairclough, D. L., Butler, R. W., Noll, R. B., Dolgin, M. J., et al. (2002). Problem-solving skills training for mothers of children with newly diagnosed cancer: A randomized trial. *Journal of Developmental and Behavioral Pediatrics, 23*(2), 77-86.

Santacroce, S. (2003). Parental uncertainty and posttraumatic stress in serious childhood illness. *Journal of Nursing Scholarship, 35*(1), 45-51.

Schultz, C. L., Kemm, M. A., Bruce, E. J., and Smyrnios, K. X. (1992). Caring for fathers and mothers of children with intellectual disability: A pilot study. *Australia and New Zealand Journal of Developmental Disabilities, 18*(1), 45-56.

Schultz, C. L., Schultz, N. C., Bruce, E. J., Smyrnios, K. X., and et al. (1993). Psychoeducational support for parents of children with intellectual disability: An outcome study. *International Journal of Disability, Development and Education Vol. 40(3) 1993, 205-216.*

Schulz, R., and Beach, S. R. (1999). Caregiving as a risk factor for mortality: the Caregiver Health Effects Study. *JAMA, 282*(23), 2215-2219.

Schwartz, L., and Drotar, D. (2004). Effects of written emotional disclosure on caregivers of children and adolescents with chronic illness, *Journal of Pediatric Psychology, 29*(2), 105-118.

Scorgie, K., Wilgosh, L., and McDonald, L. (1998). Stress and coping in families of children with disabilities: An examination of recent literature. *Developmental Disabilities Bulletin Vol. 26(1) 1998, 22-42.*

Shechtman, Z., and Gilat, I. (2005). The Effectiveness of Counseling Groups in Reducing Stress of Parents of Children With Learning Disabilities. *Group Dynamics: Theory, Research, and Practice, 9*(4), 275-286.

Sloper, P. (2000). Predictors of distress in parents of children with cancer: a prospective study. *Journal of Pediatric Psychology, 25*(2), 79-91.

Steele, R., Dreyer, M., and Phipps, S. (2004). Patterns of maternal distress among children with cancer and their association with child emotional and somatic distress. *Journal of Pediatric Psychology, 29*(7), 507-517.

Stewart, J. L., and Mishel, M. H. (2000). Uncertainty in childhood illness: a synthesis of the parent and child literature. *Scholarly Inquiry for Nursing Practice, 14*(4), 299-319; discussion 321-296.

Stoneman, Z., and Gavidia-Payne, S. (2006). Marital Adjustment in Families of Young Children With Disabilities: Associations With Daily Hassles and Problem-Focused Coping. *American Journal on Mental Retardation Vol. 111(1) Jan 2006, 1-14.*

Streisand, R., Braniecki, S., Tercyak, K. P., and Kazak, A. E. (2001). Childhood illness-related parenting stress: The Pediatric Inventory for Parents. *Journal of Pediatric Psychology, 26*(3), 155-162.

Streisand, R., Kazak, A. E., and Tercyak, K. P. (2003). Pediatric-Specific Parenting Stress and Family Functioning in Parents of Children Treated for Cancer. *Children's Health Care, 32*(4), 245-256.

Strickland, B. R. (1978). Internal-external expectancies and health related behaviors. *Journal of Consulting and Clinical Psychology, 46*, 1192-1211.

Svavarsdottir, E. K. (2005). Caring for a child with cancer: a longitudinal perspective. *Journal of Advanced Nursing, 50*(2), 153-161.

Thompson, R. J., Gustafson, K. E., Bonner, M. J., and Ware, R. E. (2002). Neurocognitive development of young children with sickle cell disease through three years of age. *Journal of Pediatric Psychology, 27*(3), 235-244.

Thompson, R. J., Jr., Armstrong, F., Kronenberger, W. G., Scott, D., McCabe, M. A., Smith, B., et al. (1999). Family functioning, neurocognitive functioning, and behavior problems in children with sickle cell disease. *Journal of Pediatric Psychology, 24*(6), 491-498.

Thompson, R. J., Jr., Armstrong, F., Link, C. L., Pegelow, C. H., Moser, F., and Wang, W. C. (2003). A prospective study of the relationship over time of behavior problems, intellectual functioning, and family functioning in children with sickle cell disease: A report from the Cooperative Study of Sickle Cell Disease. *Journal of Pediatric Psychology, 28*(1), 59-65.

Thompson, R. J., Jr., Gil, K. M., Burbach, D. J., Keith, B. R., and et al. (1993a). Psychological adjustment of mothers of children and adolescents with sickle cell disease: The role of stress, coping methods, and family functioning. *Journal of Pediatric Psychology, 18*(5), 549-559.

Thompson, R. J., Jr., Gil, K. M., Burbach, D. J., Keith, B. R., and et al. (1993b). Role of child and maternal processes in the psychological adjustment of children with sickle cell disease. *Journal of Consulting and Clinical Psychology, 61*(3), 468-474.

Thompson, R. J., Jr., Gil, K. M., Gustafson, K. E., George, L. K., and et al. (1994). Stability and change in the psychological adjustment of mothers of children and adolescents with cystic fibrosis and sickle cell disease. *Journal of Pediatric Psychology, 19*(2), 171-188.

Thompson, R. J., Jr., and Gustafson, K. E. (1996a). *Adaptation to chronic childhood illness*. Washington, DC: American Psychological Association.

Thompson, R. J., Jr., and Gustafson, K. E. (1996b). *Models of adaptation*: Thompson, Robert Joseph Jr.; Gustafson, Kathryn E.

Thompson, R. J., Jr., and Gustafson, K. E. (1996c). *Psychological adjustment of parents and siblings*: Thompson, Robert Joseph Jr.; Gustafson, Kathryn E.

Thompson, R. J., Jr., Gustafson, K. E., George, L. K., and Spock, A. (1994). Change over a 12-month period in the psychological adjustment of children and adolescents with cystic fibrosis. *Journal of Pediatric Psychology, 19*(2), 189-203.

Thompson, R. J., Jr., Gustafson, K. E., Gil, K. M., Kinney, T. R., and Spock, A. (1999). Change in the psychological adjustment of children with cystic fibrosis or sickle cell disease and their mothers. *Journal of Clinical Psychology in Medical Settings, 6*(4), 373-392.

Thompson, R. J., Jr., Gustafson, K. E., Hamlett, K. W., and Spock, A. (1992a). Psychological adjustment of children with cystic fibrosis: The role of child cognitive processes and maternal adjustment. *Journal of Pediatric Psychology, 17*(6), 741-755.

Thompson, R. J., Jr., Gustafson, K. E., Hamlett, K. W., and Spock, A. (1992b). Stress, coping, and family functioning in the psychological adjustment of mothers of children and adolescents with cystic fibrosis. *Journal of Pediatric Psychology, 17*(5), 573-585.

Thompson, R. J., Jr., Oehler, J. M., Catlett, A. T., and Johndrow, D. A. (1993). Maternal psychological adjustment to the birth of an infant weighing 1,500 grams or less. *Infant Behavior and Development, 16*(4), 471-485.

Thompson, R. J., Jr., Zeman, J. L., Fanurik, D., and Sirotkin-Roses, M. (1992). The role of parent stress and coping and family functioning in parent and child adjustment to Duchenne muscular dystrophy. *Journal of Clinical Psychology, 48*(1), 11-19.

Thompson, S., Leigh, L., and Christensen, R. (2001). Immediate neurocognitive effects of methylphenidate on learning impaired survivors of childhood cancer. *Journal of Clinical Oncology, 19*, 1802-1808.

Thompson, S. J., Leigh, L., Christensen, R., Xiong, X., Kun, L. E., Heidemen, R. L., et al. (2001). Immediate neurocognitive effects of methylphenidate on learning impaired survivors of childhood cancer. *Journal of Clinical Oncology, 19*, 1802-1808.

Thyen, U., Terres, N. M., Yazdgerdi, S. R., and Perrin, J. M. (1998). Impact of long-term care of children assisted by technology on maternal health. *Journal of Developmental and Behavioral Pediatrics, 19*(4), 273-282.

Trute, B. (1995). Gender differences in the psychological adjustment of parents of young, developmentally disabled children. *Journal of Child Psychology and Psychiatry, 36*(7), 1225-1242.

Trute, B., and Hauch, C. (1988). Building on family strength: A study of families with positive adjustment to the birth of a developmentally disabled child. *Journal of Marital and Family Therapy, 14*, 185-193.

Van Dongen-Melman, J. E., Pruyn, J. F., De Groot, A., Koot, H. M., Hahlen, K., and Verhulst, F. C. (1995). Late psychosocial consequences for parents of children who survived cancer. *Journal of Pediatric Psychology, 20*(5), 567-586.

Van Dongen-Melman, J. E., Van Zuuren, F. J., and Verhulst, F. C. (1998). Experiences of parents of childhood cancer survivors: a qualitative analysis. *Patient Education and Counseling, 34*(3), 185-200.

Vannatta, K., Gartstein, M. A., Short, A., and Noll, R. B. (1998). A controlled study of peer relationships of children surviving brain tumors: Teacher, peer, and self ratings. *Journal of Pediatric Psychology, 23*(5), 279-287.

Wijnberg-Williams, B. J., Kamps, W. A., Klip, E. C., and Hoekstra-Weebers, J. E. H. M. (2006). Psychological adjustment of parents of pediatric cancer patients revisited: five years later. *Psycho-Oncology, 15*(1), 1-8.

Zebrack, B. J., Gurney, J. G., Oeffinger, K., Whitton, J., Packer, R. J., Mertens, A., et al. (2004). Psychological outcomes in long-term survivors of childhood brain cancer: a report from the childhood cancer survivor study. *Journal of Clinical Oncology, 22*(6), 999-1006.

In: Coping with Cancer
Editor: Léa K. Jacobs, pp.61-76
ISBN: 978-1-60456-213-2

Chapter II

Parental Coping with Childhood Cancer

Annika Lindahl Norberg
Department of Woman and Child Health, Childhood Cancer Research Unit
Karolinska Institute, Stockholm, Sweden

Abstract

Cancer in a child alters the life situation of the family. For the parents, it implies stressors of varying duration, predictability, and impact. In addition to concerns about the child's prospects of being cured from cancer, the strain relates to, for example, witnessing the child in pain, concerns about the child's future, the quality of care, supporting siblings of the ill child, negative employment and financial consequences, accepting the intensity of one's own reactions, and dealing with the reactions of others. Eventually, some parents must face the death of their child. Nonetheless, successfully completing treatment does not automatically imply a "happy end", since impairments due to aggressive cancer therapies, as well as to the illness itself, are relatively common. All in all, this combination of stressors, ranging from minor hassles to traumatic experiences, places a considerable burden on parents.

Through the trajectory of childhood cancer, the varying contexts of stressors sketched out above activate various psychological processes. Accordingly, the disclosure of the diagnosis of childhood cancer implies a psychological and existential challenge for a parent. Immediately after being informed of the child's cancer diagnosis, even successfully adjusting parents experience arousal, sleep disturbances, and other symptoms of severe stress. Furthermore, several events activate stress responses during cancer treatment. In addition, long-lasting and accumulating stressors can lead to the psychological and physical exhaustion of chronic stress. Once treatment is completed, the tangible as well as the existential aspects of everyday life need to be re-established. Moreover, parents who lose their child will be subject to grief that for a period dominates life.

Permanent psychiatric problems are rarely seen in parents of children with cancer. Nevertheless, even temporary stress can have negative effects for the parents themselves and for their children. Thus, many parents are likely to benefit from professional support interventions, brought into line with the specific psychological processes involved. This chapter outlines parental stressors, demands, challenges and burdens of childhood cancer, exemplifying the processes that may follow.

Introduction

For the cancer patient, the ability of family members and caregivers to handle their own distress is always important. This is especially true as regards parents in the paediatric care. Particularly younger children are dependent on their parents for instrumental as well as emotional support. During cancer illness and treatment, the dependency is amplified and the role of the parent becomes even more critical. In addition, a working rapport between the parents and the hospital staff is crucial for a smooth progress of the medical treatment, and for the child's well-being. Therefore, it is vital to understand the situation of the parents when a child is diagnosed with cancer.

Cancer in a child alters the entire life situation of the family. Starting from the initial shock of the cancer diagnosis, it implies stressors of varying duration, predictability and impact for the parents. As regards to the psychological challenge parents face in childhood cancer, four broad contexts are discerned. First of all, there is the mere *diagnosis of cancer*, a potentially lethal disease, in one's child. The second context is the period of medical *treatment* aiming to cure the child. During this period intensive treatment brings forth a range of short and long-term side effects, demands parents' collaboration, and loads up the daily life with treatment related concerns. For families where treatment is successful, the third framework of parental stressors begins as treatment ends. This is associated with *survivorship* and the construction of a new reality after the cancer experience. However, despite advances in the cancer treatment a cure is still by no means certain. A number of parents come up against the dreadful experience of a disease too aggressive, the failure of curative treatment, and the subsequent death of their child. In other words, the fourth possible context in the parental experience of childhood cancer is the extensive process of *bereavement*. Although they overlap and interfere with each other, each of these four contexts involves stressors with certain specific meaning. In this chapter the many different burdens of diagnosis, treatment, survivorship, and bereavement are exemplified. In connection to each of these themes is a brief discussion about various psychological processes that come about in the wake of these challenges. The examples mainly come from Western society, and can partly be comparable to the situation in other cultural contexts and in developing countries.

The Diagnosis of Childhood Cancer

The first cancer-related stressor parents encounter is the disclosure of the diagnosis. For some of the parents whose children prove to be afflicted by cancer, the information is completely unexpected. Others have suspected that something was wrong, and may have gone through a history of worry, uncertainty and misunderstandings in the medical service (Clarke and Fletcher, 2004). However, learning about the diagnosis of cancer in one's child is, for most parents severely stressful. At times referred to with euphemisms like "the big C", the word *cancer* has connotations far more dreadful than the name of diseases such as heart defects or meningitis, notwithstanding their lethal potential for children. Although the prognosis of most childhood cancer subtypes has been substantially improved, the statistical survival rates do not give assurance of the prognosis in an individual case. Therefore, a parent's fear is certainly reasonable. In the end, for the individual family the probability of survival always turns out to be 100% or 0: to survive or not to survive. Briefly, the stress of learning the cancer diagnosis originates in uncertainty about the child's survival.

Dealing with the Diagnosis

The intra-individual process that arises after learning about the child's diagnosis can be described in various ways by various theoretical frameworks. Based on crisis theory the time-course of parental reactions to childhood cancer has been interpreted by way of a linear model with discrete stages (Clarke-Steffen, 1993). After the shock associated with the disclosure of the diagnosis -- producing a "limbo" of denial, grief, anxiety and disorganization -- attention is being focused. Finally, stability is reached in a new understanding of everyday life, where uncertainty about the child's survival is a present reality. However, in the theory of crisis process we have seen a change from the assumption of a universal pattern of phases towards recognition of vast individual variations, including the importance of contextual factors.

The reactions following a traumatic event such as being told of a child's cancer diagnosis have also been described within the framework of cognitive information processing (e.g. Joseph and Linley, 2006). According to this perspective, a traumatic experience imposes information about the world incongruent with the person's worldview. The subsequent processing of the traumatic information involves alternating phases of accommodation and assimilation, where accommodation requires people to change their worldviews, and assimilation entails a reinterpretation of the information to fit the existing models of the world. These processes also relate to the intrusive cognitions, and deliberate or automatic avoidance, which are frequently experienced following a psychological trauma.

For a few parents, the experience of the crisis exceeds his or her resources, bringing about negative effects in the form of persistent psychiatric states. Indeed, learning that one's child has a life-threatening disease is recognized as a potentially traumatic stressor which, in unfavourable cases, can result in acute stress disorder or, in the long run, post-traumatic stress disorder (PTSD; American Psychiatric Association, 2000). However, although the disclosure of the child's diagnosis is a discernible traumatic event, essentially the trauma seems to be quite diffuse, relating to the threat of death rather than to any discrete critical event. PTSD associated with a child's cancer diagnosis is expressed through the three symptom clusters of intrusive and distressing thoughts about the child's disease, avoidance, of reminders relating to the disease, and an increased general arousal. For some decades, there has been a marked interest in not only detecting cases of PTSD, but also applying a subclinical model of post-traumatic stress (PTS) on the childhood cancer situation (e.g. Stuber, Kazak, Meeske, and Barakat, 1998). In a number of studies, symptoms of intrusions, avoidance and arousal have been surveyed in parents of children with cancer. However, by definition, PTS symptoms are distinguishable from symptoms of acute stress not until the stressors have disappeared. Since the treatment phase is presumed to include severe stressors, research focusing on PTS symptoms in parents of children with cancer mainly involves parents of survivors. For a continued discussion about post-traumatic stress among parents of children with cancer, see the section *Survivorship* below.

Regardless of the theoretical explanation, strong reactions are expected in parents at the disclosure of their child's cancer diagnosis and for some time thereafter. Efficient resources and successful coping efforts help parents to maintain some stability through the crisis process. When the impact of the crisis does not exceed the resources, eventually parents are able to return to former level of functioning. If circumstances are favourable, a psychological and existential challenge such as cancer in one's child can even lead to positive development (Barakat, Alderfer, and Kazak, 2006). To describe this, the term adversarial growth is used; an umbrella term comprising the concepts post-traumatic growth, stress-related growth, perceived benefit, and thriving. In line with cognitive information processing theory, accommodation has the possibility to promote adversarial growth, while assimilation may leave the person vulnerable to retraumatization in the future.

In summary, the disclosure of the child's diagnosis is generally perceived as a traumatic event. However, unlike most other traumatic events, it has to some extent a positive context: the diagnosis indicates that the "enemy" is found and defined, and can now be fought. For some parents, the trauma is accompanied with feelings of relief.

Childhood Cancer Treatment

Among the stressors of cancer treatment, the one primary concern for the parents is the cure of their child. However, they encounter several other sources of strain during this period. Most of the parents want to learn about the various aspects of treatment, and they are frequently encouraged to serve as a health care resource. Concerned about their child's wellbeing, parents closely monitor the quality of medical care, and from time to time their confidence in care is challenged as they find reason for criticism (Clarke and Fletcher, 2004; Lozowski, Chesler, and Chesney, 1993). Since the parents have a legal responsibility for the child's health, they are requested to take part in the decisions about treatment. However, confused at the quantity of complex information, and without true knowledge about the options, parents may perceive participation in critical decisions distressingly difficult (Stewart, Pyke-Grimm, and Kelly, 2005). Thus, although parents wish to have control over such judgements, many prefer to have a collaborative or even passive role instead of feeling responsible for the final decision about the child's treatment.

Medical treatment for most childhood cancers has become more effective but also more aggressive. The powerful treatment has to be balanced against unwanted short and long-term side effects. Procedures for administering treatment are developed with the intention of causing as little worry and pain as possible. Yet, children in cancer treatment often consider treatment procedures severely distressing, and treatment side effects can cause the child a great deal of suffering. Moreover, the treatment brings changes in appearance – e.g. hair loss, obesity – which, albeit temporary, older children and teenagers perceive as very stressful. Different treatment modes involve different stressors, with bone marrow transplant (BMT) being one of the most arduous. BMT is extremely taxing for the child, and certain side effects from the treatment are life-threatening. Parents face an important task in supporting their child through the fear, pain and distress associated with illness and treatment (Cline et al., 2006). They may claim to judge their child's pain better than professionals, and request more efficient pain treatment (Ljungman et al., 1999), yet parents are still dependent on the medical staff for relief of the child's pain. Thus, watching the child suffer without being able to relieve the distress is one of the primary areas of parental stressors during childhood cancer treatment.

In the face of childhood cancer and its treatment, parenting is not as easy as before. The parenting burden is generally increased (Steele, Long, Reddy, Luhr, and Phipps, 2003), e.g. children with cancer frequently display problematic behaviour (Svavarsdottir, 2005). At the same time, there is a tendency among parents to spoil the ill child and to be over-protective (Hillman, 1997). Throughout the treatment phase, the ill child typically remains the family priority (Leavitt et al., 1999; Lindahl Norberg and Green, 2007). As a consequence, healthy siblings of the patient are at risk of being neglected (Houtzager, Grootenhuis, Caron, and Last, 2004). Although parents try to counterbalance as the best they can, the task may be unachievable and they have to accept siblings expressing a legitimate feeling of being left out.

Generally, the relationships within the family are strained, and several couples experience marital discord, especially during the initial phase of treatment. Extra-familial relationships are likely to involve valuable resources, but the available support from friends often wanes as time passes (Wijnberg-Williams, Kamps, Klip, and Hoekstra-Weebers, 2006). Besides, social interactions are sometimes a source of stress, e.g. in the form of negative reactions of others.

A parent's active participation in an intense treatment scheme can also influence his or her everyday life by restricting autonomy, decision latitude, and control. In the light of the uncertainty of outcome, parents live in the present, adjourning thoughts about the rest of life and the future. As a result, the day-to-day management of additional chores and tasks may be neglected. For parents in employment, the added responsibilities and the disruption of daily life impair work capacity and amplify work stress (McCaffrey, 2006). In addition, many parents are subjected to negative vocational and financial consequences during their child's cancer treatment (Eiser and Upton, 2007).

Undergoing the Treatment Phase

As exemplified above, the strain of the active treatment phase involve a large quantity of varying demands and concerns. Coping with this range of stressors includes several different processes. To begin with, the massive accumulation of various stressors and demands interfere with the crisis processing of learning about the diagnosis. Moreover, the responses to the stressors of cancer treatment can be structured in two categories: acute stress and chronic stress.

The term acute stress is here used to denote immediate stress responses (not to be confused with the psychiatric state of acute stress disorder, ASD). Certain individual events associated with the cancer treatment are perceived as particularly distressing by a majority of the parents. For example, accompanying the child at the hospital, the parent is forced to be a helpless onlooker while the child undergoes painful treatment procedures. Additionally, in the course of treatment many parents are exposed to the experience of a sudden deterioration of the child's medical condition. Although not necessarily leading to a veritable syndrome of ASD or PTSD, such incidents certainly elicit a stress response.

When stressors are severe during childhood cancer treatment, parents' acute stress reactions include feelings of uncertainty, helplessness and worry associated with the child's disease, as well as psychosomatic and physical distress symptoms. Sleep disturbances can be an effect of caregiver demands requiring nightly tending, but they can also be stress reactions. Moreover, sleep deprived persons are more vulnerable to stress, and less able to cope with the stressors they are exposed to (Ekstedt et al., 2006). Anxiety, a core symptom of severe stress, is considered a reaction to perceptions of threat. Evidently, in childhood cancer treatment, parents have every reason to ponder serious threat. During the first months of treatment parents are likely to experience elevated levels of anxiety, as compared to parents in the general community (Sawyer, Antoniou, Toogood, Rice, and Baghurst, 2000; Sloper, 2000). However, anxiety usually recede and is within a year or so comparable to the levels reported by parents of healthy children. Accordingly, acute stress reactions occur most frequently during the first period after the disclosure of the diagnosis. Nonetheless, acute reactions to severe stressors may indeed be experienced at any point in time throughout the period of active treatment.

However, stressors do not have to be severe to have high psychological impact. Even low-intensity stressors are likely to create a severe effect, if they are long-lasting or recurrent. Each exposure to such a stressor may constitute a minimum of threat, but if the strain persists, the effect accumulates over time, possibly leading to exhaustion. Chronic stress is most often associated with excessive demand, although it can arise from other persistent conditions such as threat, uncertainty, or restriction of choice. Such stressors typically have longer time course than traumatic events. However, singly each stressor need not persist for long, as cumulative effects have been suggested to occur across different stressors (Singer and Davidson, 1986). Chronic stress responses and acute stress responses seem to differ qualitatively. For example, the endocrine activation associated with responses to prolonged strain seems to be somewhat different from the "fight-or-flight" response of the acute stress. During childhood cancer treatment the aggregate of stressors has considerable potential to entail chronic stress for the parents. Neuroendocrine measures, although rare in the study of childhood cancer parents, indicate effects which are usually associated with chronic stress (Miller, Cohen, and Ritchey, 2002). Parents' single-mindedness, with the child's cure being the one and only goal, may bring a sense of energy. However, as treatment proceeds, the consequences of chronic stress become marked, particularly in the form of physical and psychological exhaustion (Jackson et al., 2007).

In summary, the cancer treatment implies an intense phase producing uncertainty, anxiety and exhaustion. However, often parents do not give themselves space to let their reactions out during this period.

Childhood Cancer Survivorship

When treatment has been successful and is completed and no cancer cells can be detected, families enter a state that may be called *survivorship*. Several of the stressors that have dominated the everyday life up to then fade at the end of treatment. Nonetheless, survivorship is generally not free from demands and strains related to the cancer. Some concerns remain, and new are added.

Most children are weak from the taxing treatment, and the need for recovery extends after discharge (Stam, Grootenhuis, Brons, Caron, and Last, 2006). One general concern for the parents during this period is supporting and motivating their child in training and recovery. Food and nourishment become critical issues. Although caring for the child during recovery is not as demanding as the active treatment, it requires time and commitment. At the same time, support from the hospital is not as accessible as during active treatment (Jackson et al., 2007). Furthermore, successfully completed treatment does not automatically imply a return back to "normal". In contrast to the transient episode of recovery, some parents have to accept that their children are disabled for life. Impairments due to aggressive cancer therapies, as well as to the illness itself, are relatively common. The sequelae refer to problems with motor function, endocrine function and growth, infertility, obesity, cosmetic defects, just to mention a few (Alvarez et al., 2007; Duffner, 2004). However, maybe the most troublesome sequelae refer to the deficits in neurocognitive performance, including problems with memory and attention, which are particularly common among survivors of brain tumours (Duffner, 2004; Mulhern, Merchant, Gajjar, Reddick, and Kun, 2004). Such sequelae often lead to trouble with everyday tasks such as school performance and social life. When growing up, a substantial minority of the survivors run the risk of limitations in their lives regarding, for example, the prospects of finding a partner and starting a family, and socioeconomic and occupational options (Anderson, 2003; Mulhern et al., 2004). Impairment of the prerequisites for a good quality of life is reflected by demographical data, as well as by reports from parents (Carpentieri et al., 2003; Löf, Forinder, and Winiarski, 2007). Remarkably enough, parents generally estimate a poorer quality of life of the survivors than the survivors do themselves. This discrepancy may imply that parents have a wider awareness of the sequelae and the restrictions of the child's life. Particularly regarding younger children, concerns about the future is an issue for the parents rather than for the children themselves.

The ultimate extent of sequelae is difficult to determine at an early stage. Many childhood cancer survivors are spared from remaining neuropsychological and physical impairment; yet, parents of those children may still have ongoing worries about their child's continued well-being, and feel the threat of possible upcoming problems on the horizon. Then again, while parents are aware of potential setbacks in several different areas, almost certainly the most feared threat to the child's future is the threat of recurrence of the cancer, as phrased by Koocher's and O'Malley's (1981) now classical expression *The Damocles Syndrome*.

Child-rearing practices are influenced by the survivor's needs and state of health, but also by the cancer experience, which tend to make parents consider their child to be physically fragile. Parents try to live up to quite intense demands for care, with the consequences of a possibility to deepen the attachment with the child, as well as being overprotective (Hillman, 1997). Accordingly, survivorship frequently brings about changes in the family dynamics. This especially affects siblings of the survivor (Houtzager et al., 2004). In addition to worries regarding their brother or sister, they often have to carry additional responsibilities in the family, and face inequalities in relation to the survivor. Siblings' reactions include strong and dissonant emotions such as fear, anger, isolation, jealousy, shame and guilt. At the same time they face decreased physical and emotional availability of the parents, due to parents' stress and the survivor's added needs. For the parents, this situation entails feelings of shortcomings and remorse. In addition, and on top of the worry about their children, many parents meet substantial transformations of their own lives, including concrete changes as well as an altered way of viewing life. For some, this shift of perspective includes contemplating the options and decisions in life, and questioning what one actually wants to do (Lindahl Norberg and Green, 2007).

Handling Survivorship

As the childhood cancer trajectory proceeds, protracted processes are layered. Thus, the traumatic insight into the cruelty and injustice of life merge with the draining burden of countless concerns, worries and responsibilities.

Treatment end is a longed-for event. Parents describe their initial reactions as relief and joy, but also a vast tiredness and a feeling of emptiness. As the demands made by active cancer treatment disappear, there is time for reflections and for the parents' own psychological reactions. Some time after treatment end parents typically experience a down period. Through the intense and demanding period of treatment, reactions to crisis and stress have been obscured and seem to be postponed. Thus, in addition to a number of new concerns and challenges, survivorship eventually gives space for the reactions of crisis and chronic stress.

During the past decades attention has been drawn to the fact that parents often express lingering reactions to experiences from the course of the disease, even when their children have successfully completed cancer treatment. Cognitive intrusions about the disease, avoidance of reminders, and arousal have been observed in a significant minority of parents of childhood cancer survivors, with intrusive cognitions likely to be the most prominent (e.g. Lindahl Norberg, Lindblad, and Boman, 2005). Since the three symptom clusters are included in the PTSD criteria, it is generally assumed that their presence reflects a persistent post-traumatic stress process. In line with this, parents who suffer from PTSD need adequate therapeutic support to resolve the disorder. However, findings are ambiguous regarding the rates and persistence of PTS symptoms and the prevalence of PTSD among parents of childhood cancer survivors. One possible explanation is the methodological differences between studies. Furthermore, researchers argue that a full PTSD syndrome a rare parental response to childhood cancer, and the levels of symptoms typically decline significantly from treatment end and on (Best, Streisand, Catania, and Kazak, 2001; Phipps, Long, Hudson, and Rai, 2005). It seems that when the concurrent stressors subside, so do the symptoms. Moreover, it has been questioned whether observed symptoms of intrusion, avoidance or arousal are strictly *post*-traumatic in nature, since a stress response needs not to be traumatic to include alternating phases of those symptoms.

Some address the topic by considering the childhood cancer experience a possible existential turning point, rather than within a PTS framework (Chesler and Parry, 2001; Forinder, 2004). According to this view, the existential challenge sets off an involuntary cognitive restructuring, which may be taxing and lengthy, but is expected and has a beneficial potential. However, while many parents confirm personal growth and a greater appreciation of life, this is certainly not true for all. Chesler and Parry (2001) quote one father, who said: "This business about 'coming out of it stronger' is a bit of rubbish". Furthermore, worry about recurrence of the cancer is quite pronounced for years after completed treatment, and seems to fade only slowly. Undeniably, worry about relapse and second cancers is realistic. Accepting that there is a substantial threat, and yet retaining faith in life is a condition of adversarial growth.

In addition to reactions relating to extremely challenging stressors, treatment end gives room to recognize the exhaustion from the persistent load of treatment. Although yet not thoroughly studied, it appears that the emotional and physical fatigue, which often interfere with parents' efforts to recover everyday life after a child's cancer resembles the symptoms of burnout (Lindahl Norberg, 2007). The burnout syndrome, a consequence of longstanding stress exposure, is a constellation of symptoms including physical, emotional and cognitive exhaustion. Originally regarded as exclusively an effect of work stress, there is an increasing tendency to regard burnout as a potential consequence of long-term stress irrespective of its source. If stressors persist, professional support may be necessary for recovery from such stress-related exhaustion.

Then again, survivorship involves not only reactions to previous stressors. When cancer treatment is successfully completed, and the families are supposed to return back to a normal everyday life, several current issues obstruct the progress of normalization. Concerned to do the right thing, but not receiving professional guidance, parents feel uncertain and inadequate regarding the recovery and rehabilitation of the child (Lindahl Norberg and Green, 2007; Lindahl Norberg and Steneby, manuscript submitted for publication). Uncertainty particularly accompanies the adjustment to a life with a child who has long-term sequelae from the illness and its treatment. Parents generally have little opportunity to know exactly how to best support the child's development and improvement. Related to this is the difficulty of knowing which problems are challenges that should be met, on one hand, and which problems are *fait accompli* to be reconciled with, on the other. What can be improved with training, and what has to be accepted? In addition to feeling uncertainty, parents have to assimilate a new view of life including certain limitations for themselves, as well as for the child. Permanent sequelae arouse parental grief at the child's lost future, and at losing the child as he or she was. Such grief typically triggers guilt and shame. Accordingly, striving to accept the "new" child may be accompanied by a mixture of strong feelings.

Although parents are happy that the child has survived, and many feel a greater appreciation of life, this is not uncomplicated. The delight at the treatment outcome is dimmed by concerns about the future and the present. Survivorship entails a polarity with the wonderful cure from cancer on one hand, and on the other hand the tragedy of remaining impairment and the awareness of the threat of relapse. Feelings of guilt arise along with grief at changes in the child, or when not managing to just be happy. Accordingly, this polarity has the potential to produce cognitive dissonance, and parents find the conflict difficult to resolve, possibly because both sides involve strong emotions.

Presumably an effect of the existential crisis, the cancer experience often serve as an eye-opener, and bring forth a new understanding of everyday life. Parents emphasize the importance of seizing the day and living in the present. At the same time, personal achievements, such as career at work, may become less imperative. Instead, the family's well-being is the essential thing. For some, this shift of perspective includes contemplating the options and decisions in life, and questioning what one actually wants to do. The broadened as well as deepened existential perspective often gives an ability to relax as regards the minor obstacles in life. The downside of this can be a sense of loneliness, a feeling that people who do not share this experience do not really understand.

Concisely, for parents, survivorship involves working through the crisis and reappraising the view of life, convalescing from physical and psychological exhaustion, seeking to learn the needs of the survivor child, and striving to accept a world with new restrictions and threats. These are all processes that eventually resolve if the conditions are favourable.

Bereavement

Notwithstanding the progress in medical technology, a cure for childhood cancer is still by no means certain. Eventually, some parents must face the death of their child. When the grim perspective is established, anticipation of the coming death of the child eclipses everyday life. However, the final loss of the child is not the only stressor throughout this period. When cure is no longer within reach of hope, the child receives treatment aiming at symptom control and pain management. Similar to the phase of curative treatment, several chores and practical tasks are the parents' responsibility. Parents serve as spokespersons, coaches, advocates, and primary problem-solvers for the child. Maybe even more difficult than during curative treatment, parents are requested to take part in treatment decisions. Moreover, supporting the child when he or she is worried and fearful is challenging. During the final weeks and months of life, children with terminal cancer experience various distressing symptoms, for example fatigue, pain, dyspnea, fevers and gastrointestinal symptoms. Aggressive dosing of analgetic drugs is sometimes needed to alleviate the pain. The balance is difficult to achieve sufficient analgesia without excessive impairment of the patient's consciousness. In addition, the period of terminal cancer also includes demands that are only indirectly related to the illness, such as financial difficulties and the competing needs of healthy siblings, among other things. When finally the end comes, despite foreseen, and sometimes even recognized as a relief for the child himself or herself, death and the final loss of the child is a most severe adversity for a parent.

Facing Bereavement

Parents who finally lose their child to the disease have covered a long or a short way to meet this sad end. Some have hardly had the time to comprehend the diagnosis, while other families have experienced a long time of alternating hope and despair. Others again have established a survivor-identity before a malevolent relapse occurs.

During the treatment of terminal cancer parents are exposed to acute and chronic stress similar to the processes during curative treatment. Moreover, conflicting feelings of hope and grief accompany the stress. For a period the child can feel well and look quite healthy, even though it is recognized that curative treatment has failed. When knowledge of the approaching tragedy is not supported by personal experience, genuine understanding of the situation can be obscured. Furthermore, parents usually keep a grain of hope right up to the end. They often work hard at motivating the oncologists to continue curatively directed treatment, and searching for possible alternatives (Bluebond-Langner, Belasco, Goldman, and Belasco, 2007).

Indeed, it may be appropriate for parents not to surrender completely to the thought of losing their child, in order to limit a possible anticipatory grief. The phenomenon anticipatory grief, which refers to a process of accommodating to the loss of a loved one in advance of the event, is subject to certain debate; e.g. it has been argued that actual anticipatory grief rarely occurs (Corr, Nabe, and Corr, 1997). Furthermore, anticipatory grief is regarded beneficial to some extent, as a preparation for the impending bereavement (Rini and Loriz, 2007). It is known that unexpected death put relatives at increased risk of post-traumatic reactions and adjustment difficulties. In addition, awareness of the situation may help enhancing efforts to find the best possible way to spend the remaining time together. However, grieving in advance does not seem to reduce the amount of grief after an expected loss (Corr et al., 1997). Moreover, anticipatory grief is considered to involve a risk for detachment that affect the dying child negatively, and leave the bereaved parents with senses of guilt and feelings of having abandoned the child. Anticipatory grief has also been understood as closely connected to hopelessness.

Concisely, during the period from discontinuing curative treatment and until the child's death, parents waver between the two parallel processes of hope and despair, as they have to realize that death seems to be inescapable, and yet maintain some optimism. It is regarded desirable for parents to talk to their dying child about death, and from time to time hospital staff encourages parents to do so. However, when parents strive to maintain hope, they do not always feel prepared for a conversation about death with their child (deCinque et al., 2006).

When a child eventually dies from cancer, the period of psychological pressure on the parents ends, and a new phase starts. During this phase reactions to new stressors as well as exhaustion following long-term strain may be present, but those reactions are typically overshadowed by the grief. It has been assumed that bereavement is likely to result in an excessively intense and prolonged grief process if it entails a shattering of fundamental assumptions about the world (Janoff-Bulman, 1992). Indeed, the loss of a child is generally considered to be the worst imaginable event for a parent, and the grief that follows may for a period bring about significant impairment in social or occupational functioning. Grief is an individually unique experience involving a range of emotions, as for example anger, guilt, loneliness, anxiety, and emptiness, as well as tangible physical pain. Besides, the emotion most often associated with grief is depression. Uncomplicated grief can even be considered as a functional depression, with the purpose to economize on strength for the processing of painful experiences and existential challenges, and for the adaptation to altered conditions. The theoretical models of the grief process correspond to those outlining the crisis process (see the section *Dealing with the diagnosis* above). Consistent with the alternating accommodation and assimilation are the loss-oriented and restoration-oriented modes (Stroebe and Schut, 2001). These modes imply confronting the feelings of grief and the loss, alternating with efforts to focus on the current daily life and the future.

In addition to intra-individual dynamics, the grieving process is influenced by contextual factors, of which the relationship with the other parent is one of the most crucial. Thus, although both parents suffer deeply, dissimilarities in their reactions may add to individual distress, for example when their phases of loss-oriented and restoration-oriented modes disagree. However, the vast variability in response to loss implies that an array of factors influences the process of grieving in various ways for the individual parent. Likewise, the substantial individual variation regarding the expression of emotions that can be observed does not necessarily imply that the grief process is more or less adaptive.

Gradually, the family context is restructured as the parents adapt to the loss. Nonetheless, although parents function adequately and the actual grief has subsided, thoughts about the deceased child may still be central to their daily functioning after several years (deCinque et al., 2006). Moreover, a fraction of the parents experience traumatic or complicated grief, i.e. persistent intense separation distress, disbelief, avoidance of reminders, and recurrent intrusive images or dreams. The core expressions of complicated grief involve symptoms relating to both traumatic distress and separation distress, and it has been discussed whether complicated grief is similar to or distinct from PTSD. Yet, on the other hand, grief can eventually lead to adversarial growth. Accordingly, for some parents the grief process gives rise to a perception of positive personal changes regarding, for example, compassion, forgiveness, and tolerance (Riley, LaMontagne, Hepworth, and Murphy, 2007).

Conclusion

Research on parental response to cancer in a child demonstrates that the childhood cancer experience influences the life of families in a range of ways, and for an extended period of time. This highlights the importance of thinking about parental coping with childhood cancer in frameworks other than those based on a linear coping process on the subject of one specific event. Considering the numerous stressors and challenges, several types of reactions are likely to occur. Consequently, adaptation to childhood cancer cannot be expected to simply mean the absence of distress. On the contrary, the expected and adequate reactions include various aspects of distress, and distress does not necessarily imply a poor adaptation.

Immediately after being informed of the child's cancer diagnosis, even successfully adjusting parents are likely to experience arousal, sleep disturbances, and other symptoms of severe stress. Likewise, feelings of uncertainty, anxiety etc. are reasonable during treatment, when medical factors set the rules for everyday life. Once treatment is completed most parents need time for recovery, as the intense feelings fade slowly. "Survivor" parents striving to re-establish the tangible and existential aspects of an everyday life can expect psychological effects of the process. Finally, for those who lose their child, grief will dominate life for a period. Such reactions are transient, and most parents end up without remaining psychiatric problems. Nevertheless, temporarily debilitating as well as long-standing stress may have negative effects on parents' health, social life, vocational career, and economy. Moreover, as a secondary effect, parental stress overload is likely to negatively influence the lives of the children. Health care professionals meeting the families should bear in mind that parents are particularly afflicted by accumulative stress during the period when the medical care system demands the most of their collaboration.

A comprehensive paediatric care model should maintain a close monitoring of parents' coping efficacy, and offer adequate support to those who need. Furthermore, continuous attention is warranted not only at the first hospital referral, but also throughout treatment and at the transition to survivorship. For the supporting clinician, it is vital to identify the nature of the individual parent's distress. For example, parents' struggling to cope with excess of current stressors as well as those showing signs of persistent post-traumatic symptoms may both be in need of professional support, although the type of interventions may differ.

References

Alvarez, J. A., Scully, R. E., Miller, T. L., Armstrong, F. D., Constine, L. S., Friedman, D. L., et al. (2007). Long-term effects of treatments for childhood cancers. *Current Opinion in Pediatrics, 19*(1), 23-31.

American Psychiatric Association. (2000). *Diagnostic and statistical manual of mental disorders: DSM-IV-TR* (4th text revision ed.). Washington, DC: American Psychiatric Association.

Anderson, N. E. (2003). Late complications in childhood central nervous system tumour survivors. *Current Opinion in Neurology, 16*(6), 677-683.

Barakat, L. P., Alderfer, M. A., and Kazak, A. E. (2006). Posttraumatic growth in adolescent survivors of cancer and their mothers and fathers. *Journal of Pediatric Psychology, 31*(4), 413-419.

Best, M., Streisand, R., Catania, L., and Kazak, A. E. (2001). Parental distress during pediatric leukemia and posttraumatic stress symptoms (ptss) after treatment ends. *Journal of Pediatric Psychology, 26*(5), 299-307.

Bluebond-Langner, M., Belasco, J. B., Goldman, A., and Belasco, C. (2007). Understanding parents' approaches to care and treatment of children with cancer when standard therapy has failed. *Journal of Clinical Oncology, 25*(17), 2414-2419.

Carpentieri, S. C., Meyer, E. A., Delaney, B. L., Victoria, M. L., Gannon, B. K., Doyle, J. M., et al. (2003). Psychosocial and behavioral functioning among pediatric brain tumor survivors. *Journal of Neuro-Oncology, 63*(3), 279-287.

Chesler, M. A., and Parry, C. (2001). Gender roles and/or styles in crisis: an integrative analysis of the experiences of fathers of children with cancer. *Qualitative Health Research, 11*(3), 363-384.

Clarke, J. N., and Fletcher, P. C. (2004). Parents as advocates: stories of surplus suffering when a child is diagnosed and treated for cancer. *Social Work in Health Care, 39*(1-2), 107-127.

Clarke-Steffen, L. (1993). A model of the family transition to living with childhood cancer. *Cancer Practice, 1*(4), 285-292.

Cline, R. J., Harper, F. W., Penner, L. A., Peterson, A. M., Taub, J. W., and Albrecht, T. L. (2006). Parent communication and child pain and distress during painful pediatric cancer treatments. *Social Science and Medicine, 63*(4), 883-898.

Corr, C. A., Nabe, C. M., and Corr, D. M. (1997). *Death and Dying, Life and Living* (2 ed.). Pacific Grove, Calif: Brooks/Cole Publishing Company.

deCinque, N., Monterosso, L., Dadd, G., Sidhu, R., Macpherson, R., and Aoun, S. (2006). Bereavement support for families following the death of a child from cancer: experience of bereaved parents. *J. Psychosoc. Oncol., 24*(2), 65-83.

Duffner, P. K. (2004). Long-term effects of radiation therapy on cognitive and endocrine function in children with leukemia and brain tumors. *Neurologist, 10*(6), 293-310.

Eiser, C., and Upton, P. (2007). Costs of caring for a child with cancer: a questionnaire survey. *Child: Care, Health and Development, 33*(4), 455-459.

Ekstedt, M., Soderstrom, M., Akerstedt, T., Nilsson, J., Sondergaard, H. P., and Perski, A. (2006). Disturbed sleep and fatigue in occupational burnout. *Scand. J. Work Environ. Health, 32*(2), 121-131.

Forinder, U. (2004). Bone marrow transplantation from a parental perspective. *Journal of child health care, 8*(2), 134-148.

Hillman, K. A. (1997). Comparing child-rearing practices in parents of children with cancer and parents of healthy children. *Journal of Pediatric Oncology Nursing, 14*(2), 53-67.

Houtzager, B. A., Grootenhuis, M. A., Caron, H. N., and Last, B. F. (2004). Quality of life and psychological adaptation in siblings of paediatric cancer patients, 2 years after diagnosis. *Psycho-Oncology, 13*(8), 499-511.

Jackson, A. C., Stewart, H., O'Toole, M., Tokatlian, N., Enderby, K., Miller, J., et al. (2007). Pediatric brain tumor patients: their parents' perceptions of the hospital experience. *Journal of Pediatric Oncology Nursing, 24*(2), 95-105.

Janoff-Bulman, R. (1992). Shattered assumptions: Towards a new psychology of trauma. New York: Free Press.

Joseph, S., and Linley, P. A. (2006). Growth following adversity: theoretical perspectives and implications for clinical practice. *Clinical Psychology Review, 26*(8), 1041-1053.

Koocher, G. P., and O'Malley, J. E. (1981). The Damocles syndrome: psychosocial consequences of surviving childhood cancer. New York, NY: McGraw-Hill.

Leavitt, M., Martinson, I. M., Liu, C. Y., Armstrong, V., Hornberger, L., Zhang, J. Q., et al. (1999). Common themes and ethnic differences in family caregiving the first year after diagnosis of childhood cancer: Part II. *Journal of Pediatric Nursing, 14*(2), 110-122.

Lindahl Norberg, A. (2007). Burnout in parents of children surviving brain tumour. *Journal of Clinical Psychology in Medical Settings, 14*(2).

Lindahl Norberg, A., and Green, A. (2007). Stressors in the daily life of parents after a child's successful cancer treatment. *Journal of Psychosocial Oncology, 25*(3).

Lindahl Norberg, A., Lindblad, F., and Boman, K. K. (2005). Parental traumatic stress during and after paediatric cancer treatment. *Acta Oncologica, 44*(4), 382-388.

Lindahl Norberg, A., and Steneby, S. Parents of children surviving brain tumour: A happy ending and a rough beginning. (manuscript submitted for publication)

Lozowski, S., Chesler, M. A., and Chesney, B. K. (1993). Parental intervention in the medical care of children with cancer. *Journal of Psychosocial Oncology, 11*(3), 63-88.

Löf, C., Forinder, U., and Winiarski, J. (2007). Risk factors for lower health-related QoL after allogeneic stem cell transplantation in children. *Pediatric Transplantation, 11*(2), 145-151.

McCaffrey, C. N. (2006). Major stressors and their effects on the well-being of children with cancer. *Journal of Pediatric Nursing, 21*(1), 59-66.

Miller, G. E., Cohen, S., and Ritchey, A. K. (2002). Chronic psychological stress and the regulation of pro-inflammatory cytokines: a glucocorticoid-resistance model. *Health Psychology, 21*(6), 531-541.

Mulhern, R. K., Merchant, T. E., Gajjar, A., Reddick, W. E., and Kun, L. E. (2004). Late neurocognitive sequelae in survivors of brain tumours in childhood. *The Lancet Oncology, 5*(7), 399-408.

Phipps, S., Long, A., Hudson, M., and Rai, S. N. (2005). Symptoms of post-traumatic stress in children with cancer and their parents: effects of informant and time from diagnosis. *Pediatric blood and cancer, 45*(7), 952-959.

Riley, L. P., LaMontagne, L. L., Hepworth, J. T., and Murphy, B. A. (2007). Parental grief responses and personal growth following the death of a child. *Death Studies, 31*(4), 277-299.

Rini, A., and Loriz, L. (2007). Anticipatory mourning in parents with a child who dies while hospitalized. *Journal of Pediatric Nursing, 22*(4), 272-282.

Sawyer, M., Antoniou, G., Toogood, I., Rice, M., and Baghurst, P. (2000). Childhood cancer: a 4-year prospective study of the psychological adjustment of children and parents. *Journal of Pediatric Hematology/Oncology, 22*(3), 214-220.

Singer, J. E., and Davidson, L. M. (1986). Specificity and Stress Research. In M. H. Appley and R. Trumbull (Eds.), *Dynamics of stress: Physiological, psychological, and social perspectives* (pp. 47-61). New York: Plenum Press.

Sloper, P. (2000). Predictors of distress in parents of children with cancer: a prospective study. *Journal of Pediatric Psychology, 25*(2), 79-91.

Stam, H., Grootenhuis, M. A., Brons, P. P., Caron, H. N., and Last, B. F. (2006). Health-related quality of life in children and emotional reactions of parents following completion of cancer treatment. *Pediatric blood and cancer, 47*(3), 312-319.

Steele, R. G., Long, A., Reddy, K. A., Luhr, M., and Phipps, S. (2003). Changes in maternal distress and child-rearing strategies across treatment for pediatric cancer. *Journal of Pediatric Psychology, 28*(7), 447-452.

Stewart, J. L., Pyke-Grimm, K. A., and Kelly, K. P. (2005). Parental treatment decision making in pediatric oncology. *Semin Oncol Nurs, 21*(2), 89-97; discussion 98-106.

Stroebe, M., and Schut, H. (2001). Models of coping with bereavement: A review. In M. Stroebe, R. O. Hansson, W. Stroebe and H. Schut (Eds.), *Handbook of Bereavement*

Research: Consequences, Coping, and Care. Washington, DC: American Psychological Association Press.

Stuber, M. L., Kazak, A. E., Meeske, K., and Barakat, L. P. (1998). Is posttraumatic stress a viable model for understanding responses to childhood cancer? *Child and adolescent psychiatric clinics of North America, 7*(1), 169-182.

Svavarsdottir, E. K. (2005). Caring for a child with cancer: a longitudinal perspective. *Journal of Advanced Nursing, 50*(2), 153-161.

Wijnberg-Williams, B. J., Kamps, W. A., Klip, E. C., and Hoekstra-Weebers, J. E. (2006). Psychological distress and the impact of social support on fathers and mothers of pediatric cancer patients: long-term prospective results. *Journal of Pediatric Psychology, 31*(8), 785-792.

In: Coping with Cancer
Editor: Léa K. Jacobs, pp. 77-93

ISBN: 978-1-60456-213-2

Chapter III

Toward Psychological Intervention for Cancer Patients: Emotional Suppression, Psychological Distress, and Coping with Cancer

***Yumi Iwamitsu**[*1] **and Ross Buck**[2]*
[1] Kitasato University, Sagamihar, Japan
[2] University of Connecticut, Storrs, CT

Abstract

Most patients facing cancer experience strong negative emotion including depression, anxiety, and sadness. They have worries including fear of death, fear of cancer, recurrence of cancer, and side-effects of treatment. Moreover, they worry about their family, their job, and their quality of life. In particular, patients who demonstrate the Type C behavior pattern including emotional suppression, and those who show higher anxious preoccupation, fatalistic and helplessness/hopelessness attitudes to cancer tend to manifest higher psychological distress. On the other hand, those who show a fighting spirit to cancer tend to experience lower psychological distress. Therefore, coping patterns under extreme stress are key factors predicting psychological distress and QOL. Our research has suggested that certain coping patterns including emotional suppression is associated with psychological distress before and after disclosure of cancer. Therefore, we proposed that patients need effective psychological intervention immediately after disclosure of the cancer diagnosis. In addition, it is important for patients to continue these interventions during the progress of treatment. The critical aspects of these psychological interventions include encouraging the expression of emotion, inducing fighting spirit, accepting negative emotions, learning how to communicate their emotion appropriately, to encourage better coping with cancer and to decrease psychological

[*] Address for correspondence: Yumi Iwamitsu, Ph.D. Department of Medical Psychology, Graduate School of Medical Sciences, Kitasato University, 1-15-1 Kitasato, Sagamihara, Kanagawa, 228-8555, Japan or E-mail via Internet to (iyumi@kitasato-u.ac.jp).

distress. In this paper we introduce our method and initial trial study of psychological intervention.

Introduction

Most cancer patients experience acute and chronic psychological distress including anxiety, tension, and depression. Some patients report psychological distress since they were tested for cancer or took the initial medical examination. Undergoing testing for cancer is itself a stressful experience for the patients because it determines whether a suspicious area is benign or malignant (Benedict, et al., 1994). Patients given the diagnosis of cancer are greatly shocked and upset. Cancer patients must consider their treatment options in this shocked condition as well as think about their job, family, and future. Even if their treatment has been chosen and initiated, patients worry about fear of cancer, recurrence of cancer, side-effects of treatment, and so on. And survivors also continue to face the uncertainties that survivorship brings: recurrence, other cancers, late effects of treatment, and the potential of a shortened life expectancy (Deimling et al., 2006).

All cancer patients are faced with this highly stressful situation. However, individual patients differ in the extent to which they report feeling psychological distress. Some research investigating these differences has examined the role of psychosocial aspects such as personality traits, coping styles, social support (Chen et al., 1996, Eysenck, 1994; Iwamitsu and Buck, 2005). In this section, we examine the relationship between psychological distress and coping to cancer, and introduce our studies. Also, we introduce some psychological interventions for cancer patients intended to reduce their psychological distress.

Psychological Distress and Coping with Cancer

Development of Studies on Coping with Cancer

Many researchers have been interested in understanding the process of coping with cancer. Descriptive studies have suggested that unconscious defenses such as denial and maladaptive coping patterns are associated with psychological distress (Meyerowitz et al., 1983). Weisman and Worden (1976) systematically studied relationships between patterns of coping and psychological distress. They found that denial, as well as passivity and acceptance were associated with greater vulnerability in cancer patients. On the other hands, Watson et al., (1984) showed that cancer patients' denial was related to less psychological distress. Results of these studies did not agree completely because there were differences in methods of assessment and in conceptualizing the concept of coping.

The Mental Adjustment to Cancer (MAC) Scale was developed as a standard and reliable measure of coping with cancer (Greer and Watson, 1987; Watson et al., 1988). Using semi-structured interview techniques, Greer et al. (1979) found that the psychological responses to cancer could be categorized into four coping styles: denial, fighting sprit, stoic acceptance, and helplessness/hopelessness. Pettingale (1984) and Pettingale et al., (1985) suggested that these coping categories to cancer relate to the probability of recurrence and prognosis of the disease.

Measuring Coping with Cancer

The developed MAC scale designed for large-scale clinical research consists of 5 scales: fighting spirit, anxious preoccupation, fatalism, helplessness/hopelessness, and avoidance (Greer et al., 1989). Fighting spirit reflects the following: (1) patients fully accept the diagnosis, (2) they use the word 'cancer', (3) they are determined to fight the illness, (4) they try to obtain as much information as possible about it, (5) they adopt an optimistic attitude, (6) they may see the illness as challenge. Anxious preoccupation reflects the following: (1) they react to the diagnosis with marked persistent anxiety and accompanying depression, (2) they actively seek information about cancer but tend to interpret this pessimistically, (3) they worry that aches and pains indicate the spread or recurrence of cancer, (4) they may seek 'cures' from various sources including so-called alternative treatments. Fatalism reflects the following: (1) they accept the diagnosis, (2) they do not seek further information, (3) they adopt a fatalistic attitude. Helplessness/Hopelessness reflects the following: (1) they are engulfed by knowledge of the diagnosis, (2) they find it difficult to think of anything else, (3) their daily life are considerably disrupted by fears concerning cancer and possibly, death, (4) they adopt a wholly pessimistic attitude. Avoidance reflects the following: (1) they refuse to accept the diagnosis of cancer and avoid using the word 'cancer', (2) they admit the diagnosis but deny or minimize the seriousness and any anxiety about it. The MAC scale measures attitudes to cancer and is a self-rating questionnaire consisting of 40 items scored from 1 "not at all" to 4 "very much so".

Relationships between MAC scale and Hospital Anxiety and Depression Scale (HADS) (Watson et al., 1988) have been investigated. The results suggest that the high anxious preoccupation coping pattern was associated with increased depression and anxiety, while fatalism and helplessness/hopelessness coping patterns were associated with increased depression.

Since the MAC scale was developed, many researchers have used it to study relationships between psychological distress and coping with cancer. Watson et al., (1991) found that adopting a fighting spirit was associated with decreased anxiety and depression, whereas helplessness/hopelessness, anxious preoccupation, and fatalism were associated with increased anxiety and depression. Other researchers have also suggested that fighting spirit is important in successfully coping with cancer. In a study of psychological adjustment to advanced breast cancer, fighting spirit was found to be associated with better adjustment (Classen et al., 1996).

Similarly, Akechi et al (1998) studied predictive factors for psychological distress in ambulatory lung cancer patients. Eighty seven lung cancer patients completed scales including the profile of Mood States and MAC scale. Their results showed that Helplessness/Hopelessness as a coping style was predictive of psychological distress. Also, coping with cancer has been related to the psychiatric morbidity among postoperative breast cancer patients. One hundred forty eight breast cancer patients were asked to complete

HADS, MAC scale, current concerns and social support. The psychosocial determinants of psychiatric morbidity were poor coping responses such as low fighting spirit, high anxious preoccupation, high fatalism and high helplessness/hopelessness (Akechi et al., 2001).

Psychological Intervention to Get the Better Coping with Cancer in Adjuvant Psychological Therapy

In these studies, it has been suggested that cancer patients require psychological interventions to achieve better coping styles to cancer and thereby improve their quality of life (QOL). Consequently, adjuvant psychological therapy (APT) was developed as a cognitive behavior treatment designed specifically to improve the QOL of cancer patients (Moorey and Greer, 1989; Greer et al., 1991). APT was based on the cognitive therapy presented by Beck (1976) which alleviated emotional disorders by identifying and correcting the maladaptive thinking. APT was focused on two crucial factors: (1) the personal meaning of cancer, i.e. how the patient perceives cancer and its implications; and (2) the patient's coping ability, i.e. what the patients thinks and does to reduce the threat posed by cancer. This therapy was directed primarily at current problems and taught the patients new coping skills.

Studies in cancer patients have revealed that psychological distress was decreased and coping with cancer improved through receiving APT. Forty four outpatients with various cancers who received APT improved on measures of anxiety, depression, fighting spirit, anxious preoccupation and helplessness/hopelessness comparing to pre-therapy (Greer et al., 1991). Similarly, a prospective randomized controlled study including 174 cancer patients found that APT produced significant improvement in the psychological distress (Greer et al., 1992), Moreover, Moorey et al., (1994) suggested that the psychological efficacy of treatment persisted up to 10 months after the end of intervention.

Suppression of Negative Emotion

Suppression of negative emotion as a coping style has also has been implicated in studies of cancer patients' psychological distress. Several studies reported that suppression of negative emotion might contribute some degree of risk in cancer prognosis (Gross, 1989). Morris et al., (1981) found that women with breast cancer were more likely on semi-structure clinical interviews to report having suppressed anger and anxiety compared with patients with benign breast disease. They developed the Courtauld Emotional Control Scale (CECS) to evaluate the extent of the suppression or control of anger, depression, anxiety and total negative emotion in daily life (Watson and Greer, 1983).

Watson et al. (1991) studied breast cancer patients' emotional distress by using this CECS, and demonstrated: 1) patients who suppress negative emotion had a fatalistic attitude toward their cancer, 2) patients who suppressed anger tended to feel helpless, 3) patients who suppressed anxiety felt higher helplesness. They proposed that these suppressive patients also should improve by receiving APT by inducing fighting spirit, encouraging expression of emotions, and supporting effective behavioural and cognitive coping techniques.

Iwamitsu et al., (2003) constructed a Japanese version of the CECS and studied relationships between the suppression of negative emotion (anxiety) and psychological distress. Their results indicated that the psychological status of breast cancer patients with anxiety expression was not altered before and after the diagnosis, while emotional distress in breast cancer patients with anxiety suppression was significantly increased after being given the diagnosis. Suppression patients indeed tended to feel more psychological distress than emotional expression patients at the first visit to hospital, after being given the diagnosis, and after discharge, but not after the surgery (Iwamitsu et al., 2005[a]). In particular, suppression patients felt more anxious, depressed and angry than expression patients. That is, cancer patients who suppress the negative emotion of anxiety experienced more psychological distress and took on a passive attitude to the cancer. As these result, they felt psychological distress higher than before. We proposed that they needed to cut this vicious circle and it was important for them to change these suppressive coping patterns (Iwamitsu and Buck, 2005). Moreover, Iwamitsu et al (2005[b]) revealed that the breast cancer patients who suppressed emotion and had chronically high levels of anxiety felt higher levels of psychological distress.

Type C Behavior Pattern

In coping with cancer, Type C behavior pattern proposed by Temoshok (1987) is an essential coping style under stress that is conceptually similar to the style of suppressing negative emotion. Temoshok defined the Type C behavior pattern as involving a "chronically blocked expression of needs and feelings" and there may also be a belief that it is "useless to express one's needs". This coping pattern is characterized as being "cooperative and appeasing, unassertive, patient, unexpressive of negative emotions (particularly anger) and compliant with external authorities" (Temoshok, 1987, p.547-551). The persons who have these behavior patterns seem to be good persons and this pattern seem outwardly to be effective in many respects, because such persons do not like to compete and prefer to settle problems peacefully. However, this coping style fails to cope with high levels of stress, and patients easily develop feelings of hopelessness and helplessness (Eysenck,1994). Renneker (1981) characterized them as being "pathologically nice." Therefore, Type C behavior pattern include (1) a tendency to suppress emotions like anxiety and anger, and a bland surface, and (2) to find it difficult to cope with stress, to develop feelings of hopelessness and helplessness, and finally depression.

Temoshok and Dreher (1992) also proposed promoting skills to modify Type C behavior pattern such as the following: 1) patients should recognize their needs and they should assert their needs, 2) they should consider their negative emotion as their good or rich humanity and should not label their negative emotion on their weakness.

Our Studies: The Relationships among Emotional Suppression, Trait Anxiety, Psychological Distress, and Coping with Cancer

We studied relationships among psychological distress and coping with cancer including emotional suppression and trait anxiety. That is, we examined whether coping with cancer including emotional suppression and trait anxiety were risk factors for psychological distress before and after disclosure, after discharge. In our studies that we have reported, after patients were assigned to either a high or a low emotional suppression group, and to either to a high or a low anxiety group, their psychological distress was compared (Iwamitsu et al., 2005[a]; Iwamitsu et al., 2005[b]). It was insufficient to examine risk factors for psychological distress during the progress of medical treatment including the surgery. Therefore, we reanalyzed these data to identify risk factors on psychological distress during the progress of medical treatment by calculating the correlations between "psychological distress during the progress of medical treatment" and "emotional suppression and trait anxiety". Moreover, we examined the relationship between "psychological distress, emotional suppression, and trait anxiety during the progress of medical treatment" and "coping patterns after discharge" to identify the predicting factors of coping patterns after discharge.

Methods

Participants

The study procedure was explained, and written informed consent was obtained from 22 female patients at their first visit to the outpatient clinic of the department of surgery, Shiga University of Medical Science Hospital from November, 1999 to January, 2002 (age: mean=54.5, range: 40-72). They attended the clinic so that biopsy and histological studies could be performed.

Measures

Profile of Mood States (POMS, Japanese Version : 1990, Yokoyama et al.,)

The self-rated POMS includes 65 items rated on a scale from 0, "not at all" to 4, "very much so" that make up six subscales: tension-anxiety, depression-dejection, anger-hostility, vigor-activity, fatigue-inertia, and confusion-bewilderment. As a global measure of affective state, a total mood disturbance (TMD) score was calculated by summing the scores on the six subscales, with vigor-activity negatively weighted.

Manifest Anxiety Scale (MAS, Japanese Version : 1957, Ohmura and Sawa)

The MAS measured the extent of chronic anxiety reactions. This self-rating questionnaire consists of 65-items.

Courtauld Emotional Control Scale (CECS, Japanese Version : 2003, Iwamitsu et al.,)

The Japanese version of this scale is a self-rating questionnaire consisting of 17 items (six items in anger suppression, five items in depression suppression, and six items in anxiety suppression) scored from 1, "not at all", to 4, "very much so" (see "suppression of negative emotion"). The original version of CECS included 21 items.

Mental Adjustment to Cancer Scale (MAC scale, Japanese version *: 1997,* Akechi et al.,)

The MAC scale was explained previously (see "measuring coping with cancer").

Procedures

The 22 patients were asked to complete the POMS, CECS, and MAS instruments at their first visit to the outpatient clinic. At the second visit, they were informed of the results of the diagnosis after biopsy and histological investigation. Then, they were asked to fill out POMS immediately after being given the diagnosis, POMS and MAC scale after discharged.

Data Analysis

We calculated each score of POMS, CECS, MAS, and MAC scale. We calculated the Pearson correlation coefficients between "POMS scores at first visit, after diagnosis, and after discharge" and "each score of CECS, MAS at first visit". Next, we calculated the correlation coefficients between "the POMS, CECS, MAS scores at first visit, after diagnosis, and after discharge" and "scores of MAC scale after discharge"

Results

Psychological Distress, Emotional Suppression and Trait Anxiety

To examine the relationship between "POMS scores at first visit, after diagnosis, and after discharge" and scores of CECS and MAS at first visit, correlation coefficients were calculated. Table 1 – Table 3 show the relationships between POMS at each session and CECS and MAS at the first visit to hospital. Results indicated that the MAS was significantly correlated with many sub-scale scores on the POMS at each session (r>.428, p<.05). The total score of the CECS was positively correlated with tension-anxiety and Total Mood Disturbances on POMS, and was negatively correlated with vigor at first visit to hospital (r>±.449, p<.05). Anger suppression was also significantly correlated with tension-anxiety, depression, Total Mood Disturbances of POMS at first visit; and anxiety suppression was significantly correlated with vigor and Total Mood Disturbances of POMS at first visit (r>±.395, p<.05). Similarly, the total CECS score was significantly correlated with tension-anxiety, depression, vigor, fatigue, confusion, and Total Mood Disturbances on POMS after disclosure (r>±.454, p<.05). Each suppression scale was also correlated with depression and confusion after disclosure significantly (r>.345, p<.05). Anxiety suppression was significantly correlated with tension-anxiety, depression, vigor, and Total Mood Disturbances of POMS after discharge (*r*>±.409, *p*<.05).

Table 1. Peason correlation coefficients for MAS, CECS and POMS at first visit

	POMS (Before Disclosure)						
	Tension-Anxiety	Depression	Anger-Hostility	Vigor	Fatigue	Confusion	TMD
Manifest Anxiety Scale	0.301	0.512 **	0.772 **	-0.301	0.765 **	0.560 **	0.661 **
Courtauld Emotional Control Scale							
Anger	0.620 **	0.403 *	0.291	-0.136	0.133	0.237	0.395 *
Depression	0.287	0.135	0.080	-0.420 *	-0.192	0.163	0.185
Anxiety	0.294	0.321	0.296	-0.556 **	0.277	0.324	0.426 *
Total	0.523 **	0.380	0.298	-0.502 *	0.108	0.324	0.449 *

*p <0.05, **p <0.01.

Table 2. Peason correlation coefficients for MAS, CECS at first visit and POMS after disclosure

	POMS (After Disclosure)						
	Tension-Anxiety	Depression	Anger-Hostility	Vigor	Fatigue	Confusion	TMD
Manifest Anxiety Scale	0.351	0.325	0.434 *	-0.301 *	0.535 *	0.428 *	0.466 *
Courtauld Emotional Control Scale							
Anger	0.530 **	0.404 *	0.230	-0.255	0.375	0.511 **	0.460 *
Depression	0.364	0.404 *	0.262	-0.418 *	0.267	0.345 *	0.415 *
Anxiety	0.366	0.431 *	0.358	-0.355	0.530 **	0.575 **	0.512 **
Total	0.552 **	0.547 **	0.379	-0.454 *	0.526 **	0.637 **	0.614 **

Table 3. Peason correlation coefficients for MAS, CECS at first visit and POMS after discharge

	POMS (After Discharge)						
	Tension-Anxiety	Depression	Anger-Hostility	Vigor	Fatigue	Confusion	TMD
Manifest Anxiety Scale	0.508 **	0.466 *	0.613 **	-0.513 **	0.373	0.603 **	0.602 **
Courtauld Emotional Control Scale							
Anger	0.244	-0.018	0.097	0.268	-0.408 *	-0.066	-0.081
Depression	-0.043	-0.115	0.020	-0.080	-0.176	0.008	-0.081
Anxiety	0.426 *	0.409 *	0.353	-0.504 *	0.259	0.539	0.478 *
Total	0.288	0.140	0.218	-0.097	-0.119	0.234	0.162

*p <0.05, **p <0.01.

Identifying the Predicting Factors of Coping Patterns after Discharge

To examine relationships between "CECS and MAS at first visit, the POMS at each session," and "MAC scale after discharge", correlation coefficients were calculated. The anger-hostility score of POMS at first visit was correlated with the Helplessness/Hopelessness score (r=.398, p>.05). The Confusion score of POMS at first visit was correlated with the Helplessness/Hopelessness score (r=.423, p>.05) (see table 4). On table 5, the POMS vigor score after disclosure was correlated with fatalism and avoidance (r>.414, p>.05). The MAC scale Avoidance score was correlated with confusion and Total Mood Disturbances of POMS after disclosure negatively (r> - .424, p>.05). On table 6, the fighting spirit score of the MAC scale was positively correlated with the POMS vigor score after discharge (r=.546, p>.01), and negatively correlated with POMS fatigue, confusion, and Total Mood Disturbances scores after discharge (r> - .433, p>.05). The MAC scale Helplessness/Hopelessness score was negatively correlated with the POMS vigor score after discharge (r= - .428, p>.01), and positively correlated with POMS depression, fatigue, confusion, and total mood disturbance scores after discharge (r>.449, p>.05). Scores of CECS and MAS at first visit were not correlated with the MAC scale.

Table 4. Peason correlation coefficients for POMS at first visit and MAC scale after discharge

	Mental Adjustment toCancer Scale				
	Fighting Spirit	Helplessness/ Hopelessness	Anxious Preoccupation	Fatalism	Avoidance
POMS (First Visit)					
Tension-Anxiety	0.016	-0.090	0.352	0.189	-0.217
Depression-Dejection	-0.181	0.149	0.381	0.125	-0.234
Anger-Hostility	-0.297	0.398 *	0.276	-0.122	-0.284
Vigor	0.282	0.024	0.062	0.045	0.184
Fatigue	-0.312	0.324	0.086	-0.077	-0.280
Confusion	-0.078	0.180	0.423 *	0.089	-0.157
TMD	-0.244	0.194	0.299	0.033	-0.287

Table 5. Peason correlation coefficients for POMS after disclosure and MAC scale after discharge

	Mental Adjustment toCancer Scale				
	Fighting Spirit	Helplessness/ Hopelessness	Anxious Preoccupation	Fatalism	Avoidance
POMS (After Surgery)					
Tension-Anxiety	0.133	-0.363	-0.218	-0.348	-0.384
Depression-Dejection	0.111	-0.065	-0.019	-0.263	-0.363
Anger-Hostility	0.010	-0.081	0.007	-0.287	-0.372
Vigor	0.323	-0.042	0.189	0.414 *	0.417 *
Fatigue	-0.128	-0.035	-0.057	-0.322	-0.367
Confusion	-0.031	0.173	-0.035	-0.120	-0.424 *
TMD	-0.044	-0.086	-0.113	-0.356	-0.449 *

Table 6. Peason correlation coefficients for POMS and MAC scale after discharge

	Mental Adjustment toCancer Scale				
	Fighting Spirit	Helplessness/ Hopelessness	Anxious Preoccupation	Fatalism	Avoidance
POMS (After Discharge)					
Tension-Anxiety	-0.170	0.403	0.145	0.107	-0.203
Depression-Dejection	-0.385	0.541 **	0.236	0.173	-0.171
Anger-Hostility	-0.307	0.349	0.290	-0.085	-0.318
Vigor	0.546 **	-0.428 *	0.111	0.174	0.288
Fatigue	-0.551**	0.465 *	-0.049	-0.235	-0.212
Confusion	-0.433*	0.449 *	0.011	-0.046	-0.173
TMD	-0.469*	0.524 **	0.132	-0.037	-0.270

*p <0.05, **p <0.01.

Discussions

Our study's aim was to identify the risk factors on psychological distress and predicting factors coping patterns after discharge. Our results revealed that (1) trait anxiety and emotional suppression were risk factors for psychological distress. Especially, anxiety suppression was risk factor for psychological distress after discharge. Our results supported the emotional suppression study on Watson et al (1991) and our past studies (Iwamitsu et al., 2003; Iwamitsu et al., 2005[a]). A high level of trait anxiety as a personality characteristic is also a key factor in psychological distress as well as Iwamitsu, et al., (2005[b]) have reported.

Next, our results founded that psychological distress before and after disclosure were the predicting factors on coping patterns after discharge. That is, if patients have higher psychological distress during the progress of medical treatment, their coping patterns might cause maladjustment after discharge. Therefore cancer patients who have higher psychological distress should receive psychological intervention to support adaptive coping patterns.

Although emotional suppression and trait anxiety did not predict coping patterns after discharge, Watson et al., (1991) reported that cancer patients with emotional suppression tend to adopt an attitude of fatalism and helplessness in relation to cancer. Temoshok (1987) also suggested that emotional suppression may be linked to helplessness or hopelessness in cancer patients. There were our two limitations which may explain why our results did not support their findings: (1) we measured the CECS only at first visit to hospital, and did not measure it after disclosure and discharge. (2) The number participant patients was small. Therefore, we continue the study to examine these points in the future.

In summary, cancer patients—especially those who suppress negative emotion, show a high level of trait anxiety, and high psychological distress—need psychological interventions encouraging them to express negative emotion, decrease anxiety, and improve coping. Iwamitsu et al., (2005[b]) proposed that disclosure of the diagnosis is a point of overwhelming stress and a critical time to intervene with treatment. We suggested that cancer patients should receive the psychological intervention immediately after the disclosure of the diagnosis. And it is also essential for them to receive genuine social and emotional support, and feedback to deal adequately with the negative and unfamiliar feelings associated with their serious illness (Reardon and Buck, 1989).

Our Trial Study of Psychological Intervention for Cancer Patients with Suppressed Emotion

We have suggested that to maintain their psychological adjustment in the face of the disease, cancer patients who suppress emotion and experience chronic high anxiety need psychological intervention including encouraging the expression of negative emotion immediately after the disclosure of the diagnosis of breast cancer (Iwamitsu and Buck, 2005). Therefore, we attempted to do the psychological intervention for breast cancer patients who suppress negative emotion on the basis of the cognitive and behavior therapy, APT, and skills to modify the Type C behavior pattern. We introduce the methods of psychological intervention and these results.

Methods

Participants and Procedures

Six early-stage breast cancer patients (age: mean=56.8, range: 42-66) received psychological interventions after disclosure, during hospitalization, after surgery, and after discharge. Their written informed consent was obtained after explaining the study procedure. They were measured the CECS instruments at their first visit to the outpatient clinic of the department of surgery, Shiga University of Medical Science Hospital from October, 2001 to February, 2003. Their score of the CECS was higher than the median value of CECS reported in Iwamitsu et al., (2005[a]). Then, they were asked to fill out the POMS immediately after being given the diagnosis, after disclosure, and after discharge.

Measures

The measures were the CECS and POMS scales used in the study previously described.

Psychological Intervention

Figure 1 shows the time schedule of psychological intervention. We asked patients to complete the POMS, CECS and so on at their first visit. Then, we met with patients who had high CECS scores immediately after disclosure, during hospitalization, after surgery, and after discharge. Each session of psychological intervention lasted 30-40 minutes. Our attitudes were consistently supportive of patients. The main skills encouraged in the psychological intervention involved cognitive and behavior therapy, APT, and skills to modify Type C.

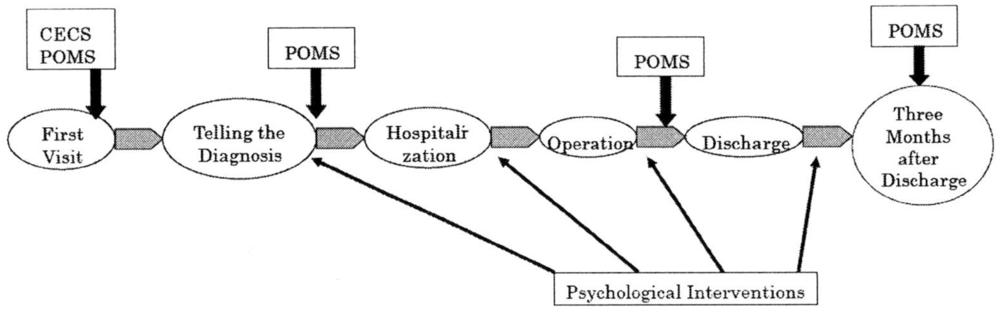

Figure 1. Procedures of psychological intervention.

After disclosure, we asked them to talk about the course of illness until they were told the diagnosis, and their current thinking and moods including fear, anxiety, etc, when thinking of their disease. As interventions we advised them with messages such as the following: (1) even though they might feel anger, anxiety, and sadness, their psychological response was the normal response of cancer patients who were given the diagnosis, (2) these emotions did not reflect their mental weakness and mental vulnerabilities (3) they should not consider anger, anxiety, and sadness as "negative" emotions, but as normal and expected. That is, we attempted to give them confidence that they should accept their emotions and express them freely.

Before surgery, we asked them to talk about their emotions and thinking before entering the hospital. As we did after disclosure, we again guaranteed that they could talk about their emotions freely, and we told them that they should not suppress their emotions. We confirmed the degree of the patients' understanding of this treatment.

After surgery, patients were asked to talk about their current thinking and emotions of disease. Sometimes we tried to modify their distorted thinking about the disease, for instance, that their life was at the end due to cancer, or that the cause of the cancer was punishment for them. And, we talked concretely about their living after discharge, especially their concerns and problems, and who they had been before having cancer. We encouraged them to modify suppressive patterns of coping.

After discharge, patients were asked to talk about their thinking and emotion of cancer since discharge. We encouraged them to tell other people of their needs, their dissatisfactions, their frustrations, and their negative emotions. They were asked to think about their coping with stress, and tell about their changed coping patterns before and after having cancer. Also, they were asked to think about the differences in their thinking and emotions before and after having cancer. Finally, we advised them that they should live more comfortably and relax.

Data Analyses

We used 12 participants who suppressed negative emotion in our past study (Iwamitsu et al., 2005[a]) as control group. Then, to comparing the intervention group to this control group, we conducted two-way analysis of variance (two-way ANOVA) [group (intervention group vs control group) × session (at first visit, after diagnosis, after surgery, after discharge)].

Results and Discussions

Figure 2 shows changes in the Total Mood Disturbance scores of the POMS in the intervention and control groups. We compared the Total Mood Disturbances of POMS on the 4 sessions between the intervention group and control group. The Total Mood Disturbances score in the intervention group was lower than that in the control group ($F(1,16)=3.37$, $p>.10$). We found that patients with emotional suppression decreased their psychological distress by receiving the intervention, although the size of the intervention group was small. The main points on our intervention were to help the patients to identify their emotion and thinking and to teach them how to communicate to others appropriately. They should not suppress their needs and dissatisfaction. Then, they had to learn appropriate coping patterns. Also, they should change the belief that suppressing negative emotion is the best way to cope with cancer (Iwamitsu et al., 2005b). As Reardon and Buck (1989) pointed out, patients who suppress negative emotion may need emotional education to learn how to communicate their negative and positive emotion accurately under extreme stress. Therefore, we did not advise patients to express negative emotions extremely, or to the exclusion of more positive emotion. In particular, we did not force them to express negative emotions. Forcing them to express their negative emotion inappropriately might actually increase their psychological distress.

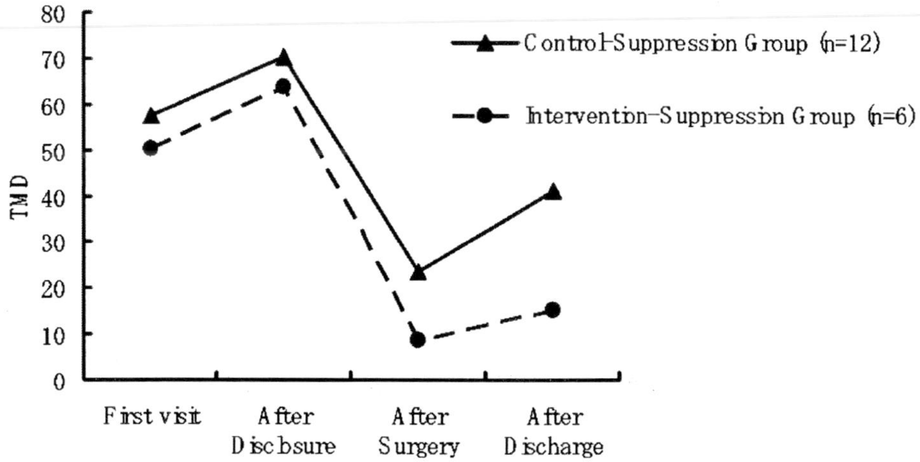

Figure 2. Changes in the Total Mood Disturbance scores of POMS in intervention group and control group.

On the other points of our intervention, we tried to accept their negative emotion, thinking, and coping patterns they have used. Our attitude was consistently supportive for patients and we told them that they did not need to deny their usual coping patterns including emotional suppression. They should accept their lives, their coping patterns, and their thinking before they had cancer. It is important for them to acquire better and appropriate coping patterns under stressful situations with having cancer from now, to have a good time and to relax in their daily lives.

Summary

We studied psychological distress and coping to cancer including the role of emotional suppression. Most patients faced to cancer feel negative emotion such as depression, anxiety, and sadness. They have worries including fear of death, fear of cancer, recurrence of cancer, and side-effects of treatment. Moreover, they generally worry about their family, job, and QOL. Particularly, patients showing the Type C behavior pattern including emotional suppression, and those who have higher anxious preoccupation, fatalism, and a helpless/hopeless attitude to cancer, report higher psychological distress. On the other hands, those who have a fighting spirit attitude to cancer report lower psychological distress. Therefore, coping patterns under stress are key factors predicting psychological distress and QOL. Recently, Bardwell et al., (2006) revealed that depressive symptoms in women treated for early-stage breast cancer are strongly linked with many subjective psychological variables; that is, coping with cancer or attitude to cancer including ambivalence over expressing negative emotion, poorer social functioning, and less optimism. Therefore, patients who have inappropriate coping patterns and distorted thinking to cancer need to receive psychological intervention immediately after giving the disclosure of the cancer diagnosis. Moreover, it is essential that they continue these interventions during the progress of treatment. We report that cancer patients who receive psychological interventions including expressing emotion, accepting their negative emotion, learning how to communicate their emotion appropriately, and getting the better coping with cancer decreased their psychological distress. Finally, these interventions based upon cognitive and behavior therapy might be effective for early-stage cancer patients as this study suggests. In the future, we hope that these intervention studies for various cancer patients will be further developed, refined, and tested on larger patient populations.

Acknowledgements

This study was supported by a Grant-in-Aid for Scientific Research, Ministry of Education of Japan(#18530543).

References

Akechi,T., Kugaya, A., Okamura, H., Mikami, I., Nishiwaki, Y., Gukue, M., Yamawaki, S., and Uchitomi, Y. 1997 Validity and reliability of the Japanese version of Mental adjustment to cancer (MAC) scale. *Japanese Journal of Psychiatric Treatment*, 12, 1065-1071.

Akechi, T., Kugaya, A., Okamura, H., Nishiwaki, Y., Yamawaki, S., and Uchitomi, Y. 1998 Predictive factors for psychological distress in ambulatory lung cancer patients. *Support Care Caner*, 6, 281-286.

Akechi, T., Okuyama, T., Imoto, S., Yamawaki, S., and Uchitomi, Y. 2001 Biomedical and psycosocial determinants of psychiatric morbidity among postoperative ambulatory breast cancer patients. *Breast Cancer Research and Treatment,* 65, 195-202.

Bardwell, W.A., Natarajan, L., Dimsdale, J.E., Rock, C.L., Mortimer, J.E., Hollenbach, K., and Pierce, J.P. 2006 Objective cancer-related variables are not associated with depressive symptoms in women treated for early-stage breast cancer. *Journal of Clinical Oncology,* 24, 2420-2427.

Beck, A.T. 1976 *Cognitive therapy and the emotional disorders*. International Universities Press: New York.

Benedict, S., Williams, R.D., Baron, P.L. 1994 Recalled anxiety: From discovery to diagnosis of a benign breast mass. *Oncology Nursing Forum*, 21, 1723-1727.

Chen, C.C., David, A., Thompson, K., Smith, C., Lea, S., and Fahy,T. 1996 Coping strategies and psychiatric morbidity in women attending breast assessment clinics. *Journal of Psychosomatic Research*, 40, 265-270.

Classen C., Koopman, C., Angell, K., and Spiegel, D. 1996 Coping styles associated with psychological adjustment to advanced breast cancer. *Health Psychology*, 15, 434-437.

Deimling, G.T., Bowman, K.F., Sterns,S., Wagner, L.J., and Kahana, B. 2006 Cancer-related health worries and psychological distress among older adult, long-term cancer survivors. *Psycho-Oncology*, 15, 306-320.

Eysenck, H.J. 1994 Cancer, personality and stress: Prediction and prevention. *Advances in Behavior Research and Therapy*, 16, 167-215.

Greer, S., Moorey, S., and Watson, M. 1989 Patients' adjustment to cancer: the Mental Adjustment to Cancer (MAC) scale vs clinical ratings. *Journal of Psychosomatic Research*, 33, 373-377.

Greer, S., Moorey, S., and Baruch, J. 1991 Evaluation of adjuvant psychological therapy for clinically referred cancer patients. *British Journal of Cancer*, 63, 257-260.

Greer, S., Moorey, S., and Baruch, J. Watson, M., Robertson, B.M., Mason, A., Rowden, L., Law, M.G., and Bliss, J.M. 1992 Adjuvant psychological therapy for patients with cancer: a prospective randomized trial. *BMJ.*

Greer, S., Morris, T., and Pettingale, K.W. 1979 Psychological response to breast cancer: Effect on outcome. *Lancet*, 2, 785-787.

Greer, S., and Watson, M. 1987 Mental adjustment to cancer: its management and prognostic importance. *Cancer Surveys*, 6, 439-454.

Gross, J. 1989 Emotional suppression in cancer onset and progression. *Social Science and Medicine,* 12, 1239-1248.

Iwamitsu, Y. and Buck, R. 2005 Emotional distress in breast cancer patients: suppression of negative emotion and social support. In Clark, A.V. (Ed.), *Mood State and Health*, New York, Nova Science Publishers, 87-119.

Iwamitsu, Y., Shimoda,K., Aiura, R., and Okawa, M. 2003 Reliability and validity of the Japanese version of the Couratuld Emotional Control Scale. *Japanese Journal of Psychiatric Treatment*, 18, 701-708.

Iwamitsu, Y., Shimoda,K., Abe, H., Tani, T., Kodama, M., and Okawa, M. 2003 Differences in emotional inhibition and those with emotional expression. *Psychiatry and Clinical Neurosciences*, 57, 289-294.

Iwamitsu, Y., Shimoda,K., Abe, H., Tani, T., Okawa, M., and Buck, R. 2005[a] The relationship between negative emotional suppression and emotional distress in breast cancer diagnosis and treatment. *Health Communication,* 18, 201-215.

Iwamitsu, Y., Shimoda, K., Abe, H., Tani, T., Okawa, M., and Buck, R. 2005[b] Anxiety, emotional suppression, and psychological distress before and after breast cancer diagnosis. *Psychosomatics*, 46, 19-24.

Meyerowitz, B.E., Heinrich, R.L., and Schag, C.C. 1983 A competency based approach to cancer. In T.G. Burish and L.A. Bradley (Eds.), Coping with chronic disease, New York, Academic, 137-158.

Morrey, S., and Greer, S. 1989 *Psychological therapy for patients with cancer: a new approach.* Heinemann Medical Books: Oxford.

Moorey, S., Greer, S., Watson, M., Baruch, J.D., Robertson, B.M., Mason, A., Rowden, L., Tunmore, R., Law, M., and Bliss, J.M. 1994 Adjuvant psychological therapy for patients with cancer: outcome at one year. *Psycho-Oncology*, 3, 39-46.

Morris, T., Greer, S., Pettingale, K.W., Watson, M. 1981 Patterns of expression of anger and their psychological correlates in women with breast cancer. *Journal of Psychosomatic Research*, 25, 111-117.

Ohumura, M., and Sawa, H. 1957, Taylor's anxiety scale in Japan. *Psychologia.*

Pettingale K.W. 1984 Coping and cancer prognosis. *Journal of Psychosomatic Research*, 28, 363-364.

Pettingale, L.W., Morris, T., Greer, S., and Haybittle, J.L. 1985 Mental attitudes to caner: an additional prognostic factor. *Lancet* ,1, 750.

Readon, K.K. and Buck, R. 1989 Emotion, reason, and communication in coping with cancer. *Health Psychology*, 1, 41-54.

Renneker, R. 1981 Cnaner and psychotherapy. In J.G. Goldberg (Ed.), *Psychotherapeutic treatment of cancer patients.* New York: Free Press.

Temoshok, L. 1987 Personality, coping style, emotion and cancer: towards an integrative model. *Cancer Surveys*, 6, 545-567.

Temoshok, L. and Dreher, H. 1992 The type C connection: the behavioral links to cancer and your health. New York, Random House

Watson, M., and Greer, S. 1983 Development of a questionnaire measure of emotional control. *Journal of Psychosomatic Research*, 27, 299-305.

Watson, M., Greer, S., Rowden, L., Gorman, C, Robertson, B., Bliss, J.M, and Tunmore, R. 1991 Relationships between emotional control adjustment to cancer and depression and anxiety in breast cancer patients. *Psychological Medicine*, 21, 51-57.

Watson, M., Greer, S., Blake, S., Shrapnell, K. 1984 Relationship between denial, delay and rates of psychological morbidity. *Cancer*, 53, 2008-2012.

Watson, M., Greer, S., Young, J., Inayat, Q., Burgess, C., and Robertson, B. 1988 Development of a questionnaire measure of adjustment to cancer: the MAC scale. *Psychological Medicine,* 18, 203-209.

Weisman, A.D., and Worden, J.W. 1976 The existential plight in cancer: Significance of the first 100 days. *International Journal of Psychiatry Medicine*, 7, 1-15.

Yokoyama, K., Araki, S., Sawakami, N., Takeshita, T. 1990 Production of the Japanese edition of Profile of Mood States (POMS) assessment of reliability and validity. *Japanese Journal of Public Health*, 37, 913-918.

In: Coping with Cancer
Editor: Léa K. Jacobs, pp. 95-105

ISBN: 978-1-60456-213-2

Chapter IV

Dialogues in Palliative Cancer Care: The Value of Responsive Evaluation to Develop Shared Understandings of Good Care

Tineke A. Abma* and Guy A. M. Widdershoven
University Maastricht, Maastricht, The Netherlands

Abstract

Responsive evaluation is a methodology in which stakeholders assess the value of care in ongoing dialogues in order to create mutual understandings and to improve the quality of care. In this chapter, we illustrate the usefulness of a particular genre of responsive evaluation, in which stories and dialogues are central. Stories – for example about the relationships between cancer patients and nurses or between family caregivers and nurses – can illuminate the meaning of everyday situations and experiences. If evaluators listen to the stories of stakeholders, and foster dialogues about these stories among groups of stakeholders, the mutual understanding and respect between the parties will enhance, and shared actions for quality improvements in care may evolve. We will show how this approach in palliative care for cancer patients can help to foster conversations about controversial issues such as resuscitation policy, patient autonomy and needs of family caregivers. Through dialogues answers to ethical questions can become shared understandings about good care, leading to joint actions to improve care.

* Correspondence: University Maastricht; Dept: Health, Ethics and Society/School of Public Health and Primary Care; Dr. Tineke A. Abma; Postbox 616; 6200 MD Maastricht; The Netherlands

Introduction

Responsive evaluation can be understood as an alternative and beneficial research model for the evaluation of practices in which stakeholders are not just information-givers, but also actively involved (Guba and Lincoln, 1989; Abma and Widdershoven, 2005). Aside enhancing the mutual understanding between stakeholders, responsive evaluation aims to use the shared understanding about good care as a learning process to improve the practical actions, for example in palliative cancer care.

In responsive evaluation the evaluator fosters a structured learning process about the issues that are of importance for the stakeholders in the evaluation setting. Collecting personal stories of the stakeholders is a method to discuss these issues among stakeholders. In this process not only opinions are investigated, experiences also are taken into account; how did the participants experience the situation and what have they learned?

We will show that a responsive evaluation approach is able to capture issues of importance in cancer care that not often are at the fore in medical evaluations. It concerns the opening of a dialogue about the resuscitation policy in a general hospital and a discussion about the autonomy of cancer patients. A third issue concerns the roles and needs of family caregivers, and their relation with oncology nurses in a general hospital.

First we present the responsive approach to the evaluation of palliative care for cancer patients in a Dutch general hospital. Then we will subsequently present dialogues about three meaningful issues in palliative cancer care: resuscitation policy, patient autonomy and the needs of family caregivers. In the final conclusion we reflect on the process, conditions and themes for further exploration.

Responsive Evaluation

Between February 1997 and April 1998 a team of two evaluators completed an evaluation of the palliative care for cancer patients in a Dutch general hospital. At the time of the study palliative care was an emerging concept in The Netherlands. In the last decade there have been many developments in palliative care in the Netherlands, such as the formation of consultation teams on palliative care and the development of special courses in palliative nursing. These developments have not been taken into account here.

The design of the evaluation in the case under consideration gradually emerged in conversation with the project group that consisted of the nursing manager of the regional hospital, the coordinator of the regional cancer institute, two nurses and an oncologist.

Responsive evaluation starts with the identification of stakeholders. In the presented case these included: patients, family caregivers – relatives who were actively involved in the caring process of their beloved - and health professionals (nurses, medical specialists and general practitioners).

In a responsive evaluation approach stakeholders, including patients, actively participate in the research process (compare: White and Verhoef, 2005; Wright, et.al., 2006; Hubbard, et.al., 2007). That is to say: they are involved in the formulation of questions, the selection of participants and the interpretation of findings. In the case under consideration informal caregivers were initially not identified as stakeholders, but during the process it became clear that it was important to include them as well given their interests.

Over the course of a year, one of the evaluators worked for 3 to 4 days a week at the regional hospital. She spoke informally with many health care workers in the hospital, but also worked for one day with a general practitioner, attended home care organizations and nursing homes with special units in the region. Given the need to be inclusive of all stakeholders the team completed 25 conversational interviews with patients, family caregivers and health professionals. One of the main principles that guided the selection of respondents was variety; the evaluators tried to gain a broad spectrum of meanings. In order to collect personal stories the evaluators followed an open conversational interview style versus the more conventional question-and-answer interview. In this evaluation collecting personal stories was one way to generate issues. The evaluators asked professionals what stood out as particularly complicated cases. When it concerned patients or informal caregivers the question *'What happened to you when you/your partner became ill?'* would often be enough to evoke a story, rich of emotions and experiences.

All the interviews were tape-recorded and transcribed in their entirety, and analyzed on specific themes, narrative structure and language. The analyses were shown to the respondents to see if they agreed with the interpretation. This 'member check' is often used to check the credibility of findings. The first phases of the evaluation process were closed with an intermediary report that had the character of a working document to stimulate further dialogues. The working document led to a working conference with a palliative consult team and a series of storytelling workshops (Abma and Widdershoven, 2005).

Sharing stories in public is not very common and can evoke feelings of fear and shame. The evaluators therefore decided to start with homogeneous groups of people who had known each other for some time. In this way the evaluators created an atmosphere in which participants felt safe and comfortable enough to talk openly about themselves, their values and opinions in the form of ideas, feelings, experiences, plans and desires. During these meetings the evaluators introduced themselves and explained the goals of the workshop. After a short reading pause everyone was invited to retell the stories in his or her own voice. The initial responses indicated what participants found important and provided a good base for illuminating the different meanings embedded in the stories. After an hour the evaluators would bring the workshop to an end.

The evaluators ended their project with a final report that was disseminated within the hospital and the region of care.

Resuscitation Policy

Responsive evaluation is appropriate to capture sensitive topics, as the following story will illustrate. One of the emerging issues in the presented evaluation project concerned the resuscitation policy within the hospital. The subject was placed on the agenda by Roland (pseudonym), a nurse at the oncology ward in the hospital. He told a story, of which a short summery follows.

> What I find troublesome is the issue of following resuscitation orders or not. Mainly because the doctors are ... [doesn't finish his sentence] In certain instances we [the nurses] wonder what we should do. Imagine, for example, that the patients get a heart attack. Every time again we have that discussion. The doctor says 'We do want to make sure that everything has been done' [to keep the patient alive]. ...[Silence] And if we ask not to follow resuscitate orders that we then will ...[Silence]. If we have to motivate time and again why we not want to resuscitate someone ... [Sigh]
>
> What happens if you do not want to resuscitate a patient, because you think it is not good to do so?
>
> Well, because you often are the one taking care of a certain patient and if you see that someone is not doing well, then you talk it over with your colleagues. Like 'Gosh, it goes very badly, does it make sense that we resuscitate her? Let us discuss it with the doctor and say I have sensed that the patient does not want that [resuscitation] either.' When it goes a bit worse you bring it up, so that it will become a subject of an open discussion. At this particular moment I have just had a very bad experience. I started in the afternoon at 3.40 pm and coincidentally we were all sitting together. A woman was severely ill, and I wondered whether or not to follow the resuscitation orders. When I brought this up my colleagues replied 'No, because the doctor wants to try the air machine and everything.' In the evening she got a heart attack and the family responded 'Fortunately, she has died', but I stood there and said 'I have to resuscitate her.' And the family replied 'She never wanted this' and then you really are standing there, 'What do I have to do now?' As nurses we have to follow the doctor's policy, so I had to resuscitate her and to change the batteries of the machine.

Roland is telling a story that he prefers to forget; it was a very stressful situation where he had to resuscitate a patient against the will of the family and her own evaluation of the situation. He has a hard time talking about the issue, painful as the event was. But the story also shows that the nurses get tired of the fact that they are always the ones who have to bring the subject to the fore. Their irritation relates to the dominance of the doctors as decision-makers, and the experience that the voices of the nurses, who are often the ones who are closer to the patient, are hardly taken seriously.

As long as a taboo rests on this subject, there is no climate to develop rules that can serve as a good guide in problematic situations. The evaluators considered Roland's story a statement that should be discussed in a broader forum to stimulate a reflection on this sensitive and controversial issue. They therefore included it in the intermediary report. Other nurses and some medical doctors recognized the moral dilemma of Roland and acknowledged that in resuscitation decisions the quality of life and the view of the patient as well as the perspective of the nurses should be taken into consideration.

We conclude that the responsive evaluation helped to identify and articulate moral dilemmas nurses encountered with the implementation of the resuscitation policy in their hospital. Their voice gained a hearing, and opened up a conversation about ethical dilemmas and the communication between patients, nurses and medical doctors.

Patient Autonomy

The second theme emerging in the evaluation process related to the experience of patient autonomy and the ideas of the nurse about this principle. The theme became subject of discussion in response to a story of a cancer patient, presented to a group of nurses in a storytelling workshop.

It concerned the story of David, a middle-aged man who had recently stopped working because the oncologist had diagnosed bowl cancer. He regularly visited the outpatient chemotherapy clinic. In the analysis of the story the evaluators focused not only on themes in the story, such as the fact that the illness affects all facets of his life, but also analyzed the language (Lieblich et.al., 1998). An analysis of the linguistic devices revealed, for example, that David was using a metaphor when referring to cytostatics as 'poison'. The term poison illuminates the meaning he endows to chemotherapy: it is very dangerous, even for the nurses, who have to wear special clothing. With this term David describes how the treatment actually feels.

His deeply personal story evoked a spontaneous discussion among the nurses of the outpatient chemotherapy clinic. The nurses appeared to have difficulties understanding his story and were shocked by the use of the term 'poison'. One of the nurses objected to this 'morally incorrect' word. The evaluators reasoned that David's story might also be controversial for the nurses of other wards, and they therefore decided to use this particular story for an organized dialogue among oncology nurses.

First the story:

> Since the diagnosis I have been operated on twice. Then the trouble started. I often have to go to hospital because I have appointments with the oncologist, the stoma specialist and the surgeon. I have a card with all the appointments and they are all mixed-up.
>
> The therapies at the clinic are intensive. I go to the room where I am given my injections. People are sitting in chairs. It's like a doctor's waiting room. Nobody says anything. You chat a bit, and now and then you make a joke. The first hour I lie on a bed. I am given a yellow fluid and salt suspension. After an hour they inject the poison. But first they have to find a vein. They have to be careful, because the poison has to go into the vein and not under the skin. Quite often the nurses have trouble finding the right vein and they take me somewhere else in the hospital.
>
> Right now I am satisfied just so long as I feel good. Some things trouble me, of course. My skin has become brittle. I also get diarrhea and social contacts are becoming more difficult. That's part of it. I can still enjoy walking with my dog, cycling and working in the garden. These are my hobbies and as long I am busy with them I feel okay.

The group of oncology nurses responded as follows to the story of David:

> Amy: 'I recognize the part of the story where the patient talks about the appointment card. I have often asked myself if patients can understand the mess. There is no logical order.'

Karen: 'He [David] accepts many things as they come.'

Paula: 'I think it is a very tragic story. Where is the sick person? He just accepts everything as if it were easy.'

Donna: 'Perhaps he is trying to protect himself.'

Paula: 'That's possible but he tells everything so passively. It makes me wonder whether this is actually good palliative care and I wonder about the quality of life when someone has no control over his situation.'

In the discussion of David's story participants focused on the (lack of) autonomy of the patient. Several nurses pointed out that David was behaving very passively. He was not well informed and had problems managing his appointment card at home. However, he did not articulate these problems or express his concerns. Almost all participants agreed that he was not in control of the situation. They found his incompetence and passive behavior strange and pitiful - someone called it a tragic story - and tried to understand it.

The conversation emerging in the workshop enabled the evaluators to respond to and to stimulate a reflection on underlying value commitments, such as the principle of autonomy. The evaluators did not bring in their own interpretations of David's story, but attempted to stimulate a deliberation about the possible meanings of his story. As Socratic guides the evaluators asked questions by taken-for-granted ideas and routines, like: Should patients always be stimulated to take care for themselves? Is this also the case when patients, like David, implicitly or explicitly prefer some support, for example, assistance with coordination tasks? How do nurses adequately attend to the suffering of patients, do have a task to teach patients how to cope with their illness? Are there situations where it is better to help patients with their daily care, so that they become less tired and have some energy left to do those things (walking, gardening) that enhance their welfare and quality of life?

David's story and these questions triggered conversations among nurses and as a result they began to consider that being attentive and caring might in some instances be more appropriate than stimulating patients to act as autonomous subjects.

The Needs of the Family

A distinguished characteristic of palliative nursing is the care of a patient's family members and close friends (Doyle, et.al., 1993). Family members often find providing care to be stressful and burdening (Higginson, et.al., 1990; McMillan, 1996; Leis, et.al., 1997; Proot, et.al., 2003). A tensed relation with nurses further complicates the situation (Abma, 2005). This is the third theme that emerged in the responsive process and became subject of ongoing dialogues. By presenting the stories of both parties – family and nurses – the tensions become visible, understandable and discussible. For the sake of clarity, the patient was too ill to be interviewed at the moment of the evaluation. After a portrait of the persons and events the stories of both parties are presented.

Portrait of the Persons and Events

Sarah was hospitalized with thyroid gland cancer. She was cared for in a medium-sized general hospital in a city in the east of the Netherlands. The couple had been married for 31 years. Both their sons are married. The couple had a strong and loving relationship.

According to Harry, his wife was a strong, passionate and assertive personality. '*Sarah has always been my mate, my friend, my spouse, and my bed partner. She was everything to me. She was a very special woman.*'

Initially the nurses thought that Sarah would be able to return home. As it was planned that Harry would take care for her on her return home the nurses trained him in the skills he would need. However, it became clear that his wife was actually too ill to go home. After three intensive chemotherapy cures the doctors confirmed their original diagnosis that the tumour was not responsive to treatment.

The tumour had spread to her back causing her intense pain. Sarah received pain therapy in a local specialist clinic but this seemed to aggravate her condition. During her time in the hospital Harry delivered much of her care. This ranged from helping her with daily routine to care that required more specialized skills. Sarah died on the oncology ward after having spent almost five months in hospital.

The Story of the Husband

> 'They said Sarah was an extremely difficult case, but that case happened to be my wife!'

Harry was keen to learn the skills he would need to take care of his wife at home, such as listening to her nasogastric tube with a stethoscope and cleaning the tracheostomy tube. To practice these skills, he actively took part in her care in the hospital. He was always near her and '*keeping an eye on her*'. His presence with his wife not only concerned being around physically to take care of practical tasks, but also included her welfare. When he found her unhappy, because she felt 'dirty', he experienced this as 'humiliating.' In Harry's opinion this was one of the examples of the nurses not being careful.

The nurses had no contact with Sarah, and Harry felt the nurses did not take the time to talk with Sarah and him about her illness and approaching end. He felt upset they saw his beloved wife as a 'complicated case.' When he saw how she got breathing problems, becoming weaker and weaker, this wore him out.

> 'I was with her day and night. The nurses did not have to do anything. I did everything. They had had enough of me. Once I broke down, and then I began to worry that I would end up in the neurology ward and that Sarah would have nobody to rely on. No one to keep an eye on her, no one to see they did not hurt her and that everything was done that should be done.'

When he attempted to bring his concerns up with the nurses Harry described himself as feeling like a '*beggar, begging for adequate care.*' He did not feel his concerns were addressed and the situation continued. Harry spoke of how his trust in the nurses faded away. And he felt ignored: '*they had enough of me.*'

The Story of the Nurses

The relationship between the nurses and Harry developed in a situation in which a high level of care was necessary. The nurses described Sarah as an extremely difficult case. There were complications related to the severity of her illness and her wishes were also difficult to meet. For example, she had wanted to attend the marriage of her son. Her choice was respected, although this required a lot of the nurses: '*we had all kinds of troubles, medical interventions, a tube for breathing, extra cures, a nasogastric tube to feed her, many, many problems.*' Sarah attended her son's wedding, but afterwards she was completely exhausted. Nurse Lilian sketches the seriousness of the situation: '*The next morning she was almost dead in bed.*'

In her descriptions nurse Rosanne emphasizes the shift in Harry's behaviour after learning certain skills:

> 'There were quite a few things that had to be done... and he had to learn them all. He wanted to learn though. Eventually – when he had learned everything – his attitude seemed to be: I know how it should be done, you know nothing.'

Training Harry the required skills meant that the nurses shared their knowledge and insights with a lay person and gradually this lay person became more and more knowledgeable. The expertise of the nurses was no longer their exclusive domain. The nurses felt that Harry was not showing sufficient respect for their special qualifications as professionals. They perceived his attitude to be arrogant and it directly affected their professional pride and honour as 'experts'.

Because Harry and the nurses had to cooperate for a much longer time than originally planned, the tensions increased. According to Rosanne this was further aggravated by the possessive and authoritative behaviour of Harry: '*He acted like: this is my world. This is my wife. If you want to do something, then you need my approval. I will tell you how things should be done.*'

That the nurses were not part of the world of the couple and how disappointed they felt about this is phrased by Rosanne as follows:

> 'Our care for the woman, you know [...], the physical contacts we had with her, were made very difficult because he was continuously with her. He was always present and well, then you are not going to go in, sit beside her and take her hand and ask 'What is going on.' He was always in-between. We just wanted [...] to be with the two of us - the patient and one of us, talking about things [...] He was always present, and well, finally you started to feel 'Oh no, there is he again!' He claimed space in such a way that you could not come in-between.'

When Sarah was hospitalised the workload was high. A small group of nurses had responsibility for a large group of patients. Four nurses were responsible for 21 patients during the day and, depending on the condition of the patients, there were two or three at night. There is no time left to recover from periods of intensive work. In this type of situation it is not easy to give good palliative care. Lilian points out that the nurses are anxious to complete their tasks and whatever is needed in the given circumstances to give good care. The hectic working situation creates, however, a tensed atmosphere, while terminal patients require a relaxed and calm sphere, according to Lilian.

Lilian notes nurses should have a different approach when dealing with this group of patients: '*You should be calm and have time for them. You should try to help them express their needs and if there are still problems you should help the patients as much as you can to solve them.*'

A genuine interest in the patient, in his or her life and family are put under pressure if certain conditions are not met.

While Rosanne links the conflict between the nursing staff and the family to Harry's dominating attitude, Lilian emphasises that individual attention and care were not always optimal because of the work-load, the large group of patients and procedures associated with the institutional setting itself. The professional care given by the nurses contrasts sharply with the personal care given by Sarah's husband. In the responsive evaluation these diverging perspectives on good care were articulated and illuminated, and used as input for organized conversations among participants. In the storytelling workshops the stories of Harry and the nurses triggered rich conversations about the relations with family members and the needs of the family.

Conclusion

Health professionals acknowledged the relevance of the project and were willing to join it. Another positive condition was the fact that powerful agents - such as the nursing manager of the hospital - were willing to share influence and power and to acknowledge the evaluation and its findings. In such a context the evaluation will engender a maximum effect in terms of heightened awareness and a readiness to improve practice.

In the project under consideration the mutual understanding between parties enhanced, and improvements on a concrete level have been realized. The outpatient chemotherapy clinic, for example, has developed and implemented a questionnaire to regularly evaluate the quality of care from the perspective of patients. The consultation team for palliative care started with the discussion of complicated cases to stimulate the structural exchange of experiences and knowledge among interested health care professionals. In these clinical meetings deliberate attention is given to non-medical aspects of care, the possibilities to enhance the quality of life, illness management, the suffering and 'tragic' aspects of cancer and the limits of patient autonomy. The consultation team is still active in the whole region; giving support and advice to general practitioners, nurses in home care organizations and nursing homes. In addition a help-desk on palliative care has been installed at the hospital. Over the years, the Regional Cancer Institute has developed courses on palliative care for oncology nurses in which attention is paid to the double role of family caregivers as 'partners' in care and 'objects' of care. All the oncology nurses of the hospital have followed these specialized courses. The resuscitation policy at the hospital remains to be a sensitive topic.

Responsive evaluation of (palliative) care for cancer patients works best if evaluators are willing to give up some of their control over the evaluation process, have a tolerance for the existence of multiple realities and ambiguity and try to foster the development of a shared caring practice.

The stories about the three subjects illustrate the possibilities of developing a shared understanding of good cancer care.

The story of Roland about the resuscitation policy in the hospital provided insights in the complicated working relationship between medical doctors and nurses, and paved the way for a dialogue about moral dilemmas that had not been discussed openly among participants in the past. Participants began to acknowledge the perspectives of the patient and nurses, and the quality of life as an important consideration in resuscitation decisions.

The story of David and the metaphors he uses capture how a treatment actually feels, and how the illness affects all facets of life. David's story and that of the nurses, and the dialogue that followed, led among the nurses to new insights and a reorientation on the priorities in care; less emphasis on the strengthening of the autonomy of the patient and more attention for the tragic aspects of cancer and the needs of support and care among patients (Widdershoven, 1999).

Finally, the story of Harry and Sarah enhanced insights in complex relations between family and nurses in the context of a 'culture of quickness.' (Andershed and Ternestedt, 1997) With these insights the nurses may assist in the formulation of the feelings and needs of family members and refocus their care – perhaps in a situation of improved conditions – to include the family instead just concentrating on the patient. More generally this raises the question how the double roles of the family – caregiver and receiver of care - can be integrated in ethical theory and how to judge whether these roles are performed in a responsible way.

A recurrent topic in all three issues – resuscitation policy, patient autonomy and the needs of family – is the complicated relation and communication between the parties engaged in palliative cancer care. The voices and perspectives of patients, family and nurses are not always adequately taken into account in decisions and actions, and hence their issues (quality of life, illness management, symptoms, constraining conditions) are not always fully acknowledged. Professional asymmetry between nurses and doctors and between professionals and lay persons (patients and family) complicates the communication.

The articulation of issues of all stakeholders and the dialogue about these issues demonstrates that a responsive approach leads to a broader and deeper understanding of cancer care and to more inclusive actions to improve the practice of care. It further shows that the inclusion of the perspectives of cancer patients, their family and nurses should be strengthened in (palliative) cancer care, policy and research. Evidence suggests that patient involvement can make policy and research more relevant, and may enhance the personal empowerment of patients, assisting them to cope with cancer more effectively (White and Verhoef, 2005; Wright, et.al., 2006; Hubbard et.al., 2007). Promising examples, like those recorded in this chapter, may help to further elaborate and implement the patient involvement agenda.

References

Abma, T.A. (2005) Struggling with the fragility of life: A relational-narrative approach to ethics in palliative nursing, *Nursing Ethics*, 12(4): 337-348.

Abma, T.A. and G.A.M. Widdershoven (2005) Sharing stories: Narrative and dialogue in responsive nursing evaluation, *Evaluation and the Health Professions*, 28(1): 90-109.

Andershed B, Ternestedt BM. (1997) Involvement of relatives in the care of the dying in different care cultures: Involvement in the dark or in the light? *Cancer Nursing*; 21 (2): 106-116.

Doyle D, Hanks GWC, McDonald N. (1993) *Oxford Textbook of Palliative Medicine.* Oxford: Oxford University Press.

Guba, E.G. and Y.S. Lincoln (1989) *Fourth Generation Evaluation*, Beverly Hills, Sage. Higginson I, Wade A, McCarthy M. (1990) Palliative care: Views of patients and their families. *British Medical Journal*: 277-280.

Hubbard, et.al., (2007) A review of literature about involving people affected by cancer in research, policy and planning and practice, *Patient Education and Counseling*, 65, 21-33

Leis AM, Kristjanson L, Koop PM, Laizner A. (1997) Family health and the palliative care trajectory: a cancer research agenda. *Canc Prev. and Control*, 1: 352-360.

Lieblich AR, Tuval-Mashiach, Zilber T. *Narrative research: reading, analysis and interpretation.* Thousand Oaks: Sage, 1998.

McMillan SC. (1996) Quality of life of primary caregivers of hospice patients with cancer. *Cancer Practice*: 191-198.

Proot IM, Huijer Abu-Saad H, Crebolder HFJM, Goldsteen M, Luker KA, Widdershoven GAM. (2003) Vulnerability of family caregivers in terminal palliative care at home: balancing between burden and capacity. *Scad. J. Caring Sci*; 17: 113-121.

Widdershoven GAM. (1999) Care, cure and interpersonal understanding. *Journal of Advanced Nursing* 1999; 29: 1163-1169.

White, M.A. and M.J. Verhoef (2005) Toward a patient-centered approach: Incorporating principles of participatory action research into clinical studies, *Integrative cancer therapies*, 4(1): 21-24.

Wright, D.N.M., J.B. Hopkinson, J.L. Corner and C.L. Foster (2006) Listening to the views of people affected by cancer about cancer research: an example of participatory research in setting the cancer research agenda, *Health Expectations*, 9, 3-12.

In: Coping with Cancer
Editor: Léa K. Jacobs, pp. 107-126

ISBN: 978-1-60456-213-2

Chapter V

Can Coping Predict Quality of Life and Survival over a Five-Year Period in Women with Breast Cancer in Anthroposophic and Conventional Care?

Marianne Carlsson[*]
Department of Public Health and Caring Sciences,
Section of Caring Sciences, Uppsala University, Sweden

Abstract

A great deal of research concerning understanding of psychological distress in women with breast cancer has been conducted within the theoretical model of stress and coping. Ways of coping with stress are often classified into two major categories: problem-focused and emotion-focused. Quality of life is a multidimensional concept that refers to a person's perceived quality of her/his physical, psychological, social and existential functioning. Quality of life could be looked upon as an outcome of coping. The aim of the study was to study the relation between coping, quality of life and survival in two samples of women with breast cancer. Another aim was to study the stability of ways of coping over time and whether it would be possible to predict quality of life and survival at a later time from coping at a specific time. The women (n =120) took part in a longitudinal study of the outcome of anthroposophic and conventional care over a five-year period. Sixty women who had chosen anthroposophic hospital and 60 individually matched women from an outpatient department with conventional care participated.

[*] Corresponding author: Marianne Carlsson PhD, professor; Uppsala University; Department of Public Health and Caring Sciences; Section of Caring Sciences; Uppsala Science Park; SE-751 83 Uppsala, Sweden; Phone: +46 18 611 3422; Fax: +46 18 511 657; E.mail: ***Marianne.Carlsson@pubcare.uu.se***

Coping was measured by the Mental Adjustment to Cancer scale and quality of life by the functional scales of the EORTC QLQ-C30 and the Life Satisfaction Questionnaire.

The women were categorised into four categories based on their MAC-scores at inclusion. The categories were called: low copers , high copers , emotional copers and fighters.

Data were collected at six times, at inclusion to the study, after 1 month, after 3 months, after 6 months, after 1 year and after 5 years. Data were collected from 1995 to 2005.

There were differences in perceived quality of life between women with different ways of coping at admission to the study. The women categorised as fighters assessed higher quality of life compared to the other women and also in comparison with Swedish women in general. There was no relation between cancer stage, time since diagnosis and ways of coping. The women in anthroposophic care as well as the women in conventional care showed the same pattern over time, emotional copers assessed lower quality of life compared to fighters and high copers. Most women changed their way of coping and that was more obvious among the women who were treated within anthroposophic care. There was no relation found between ways of coping and cancer stage, time since diagnosis, or survival.

Introduction

Perceived quality of life and survival are often used as outcome measures of breast cancer treatment. Women with breast cancer usually live many years after their diagnosis and many will die from other causes than the breast cancer. To have as good quality of life as possible is important for everyone. How quality of life is perceived is due to a number of internal and external factors. One important aspect is how a person cope with everyday stress. The present study investigates the relation between ways of coping, quality of life and survival in women with breast cancer.

Psychosocial Aspects of Breast Cancer and Breast Cancer Survival

There are a number of studies on the impact of psychosocial factors on breast cancer progression. Despite that, there is no certainty or consensus about the relation between the contributing factors or processes involved. Lehto et al (2006) investigated the relative impacts of socioeconomic, psychological, and psychosocial factors on survival in breast cancer. The 102 women who participated were 72 years old or younger. The results showed that longer survival was predicted by a long education, high socioeconomic status and minimizing-related coping, while shorter survival was predicted by emotional defensiveness, behavioural-escape coping, and high level of perceived support.

Goodwin et al (2005) found that health related quality of life and psychosocial status at diagnosis and 1 year later not were associated with medical outcome in women with early-stage breast cancer. They concluded that evidence that psychosocial status and health-related quality of life are associated with breast cancer outcome is weak and inconsistent.

Coping as a State or a Trait

A great deal of research concerning understanding of psychological distress in women with breast cancer has been conducted within the theoretical model of stress and coping formulated by Lazarus and Folkman (Lazarus and Folkman, 1984), and Lazarus (Lazarus, 1993). They define coping as 'constantly changing cognitive and behavioural efforts to manage specific external or internal demands that are appraised as taxing or exceeding the resources of a person' (Lazarus and Folkman p 141). Since coping refers to a person's ongoing efforts to manage perceived stress, adaptation to stressful events such as chronical illness may be facilitated or complicated by using different ways of coping (Lindqvist et al, 2000). Ways of coping with stress, so-called coping strategies, are often classified into two major categories; problem-focused coping, in which a person tries to change her/his situation and emotion-focused coping, where he/she tries to regulate the emotions caused by the situation (Lindqvist et al, 2000). According to Lazarus and Folkman (1984), coping is a process or a state that varies over time and in different situations rather than a trait. On the other hand, a common finding is that changes over time in ways of coping are not substantial. (Nordin, 1998).

The Relation between Coping and the Use of Complementary and Alternative Medicine and Cancer

Complementary and alternative medicine (CAM) is used by many cancer patient in most parts of the world. (Cassileth et al, 2001). People who choose CAM tend to differ from those who choose conventional medicine. A review of literature show that CAM-users tend to be better educated, of higher socioeconomic status, female, and younger but also to show more psychological problems than non-users. Studies also show that seeking alternative treatment is more common among mentally distressed cancer patients (Cassileth and Deng 2004; Risberg, 2003)

Moschen et al. (2001) asked 117 women with breast cancer about their quality of life, coping, and use of alternative/complementary medicine. The result showed that 47% reported use of alternative medicine in addition to conventional treatment. Compared with non-users of alternative medicine, the users had a more active strategy of illness coping and displayed greater religious involvement. Patients using a large number of alternative therapies tended to adopt a more depressive coping strategy.

Mental Adjustment to Cancer and Coping

Mental adjustment to cancer is defined as the cognitive and behavioral responses made by an individual to the diagnosis of cancer (Watson et al, 1988). Several studies using the MAC- scale have shown that the coping strategy characterized as fighting spirit is associated with better psychological adjustment, whereas coping strategies representative of hopelessness/helplessness, anxious preoccupation, and fatalism are associated with poor psychological adjustment (Schnoll et al, 1998).

Coping and Quality of Life

Quality of life is a multidimensional construct that refers to a person's perceived quality of her/his physical, psychological, social and existential functioning (Anderson et al, 1993). And according to a meta-analysis performed by Smith et al. (1999), the perception of quality of life is a cognitive process where several dimensions are evaluated and integrated into an overall assessment.

In several studies the relation between coping, quality of life and well being have been studied. As early as 1991, Greer (1991) interviewed 62 women with breast cancer 15 years after the diagnosis. The result showed that women with "fighting spirit" and denial were better off than women who expressed "stoic acceptance", "anxiousness" or "helplessness" as a response to their breast cancer. LaFortune Fredette (1995) interviewed 14 women who had lived at least 5 years after a diagnosis of breast cancer. The women described how they tried to adjust to the new situation by using multiple coping strategies, with information seeking, work, spirituality and family being predominant.

Lauver et al (2007) interviewed 51 women aged 34-77 with gynecologic or primary breast cancer twice about their coping strategies. The interviews took place 4 weeks and 3-4 months after radiation or chemotherapy. The women used acceptance, religion and distraction as primary coping strategies. These strategies were also rated as highly helpful.

Manuel et al (2007) asked 201 women aged 50 years or younger at diagnosis 6 months to 42 months post diagnosis. The most frequently used coping strategies were positive cognitive restructuring, wishful thinking and making changes. The women found social support to be most helpful to deal with anger and depression, whereas positive cognitive restructuring was more helpful for concerns about the future.

Ransom et al (2005) examined whether problem-focused coping strategies used by early stage breast cancer patients at the end of treatment could predict changes in quality of life six months later. Questionnaires were distributed to 146 women twice. The result showed that the women who focused more on their symptoms at treatment end experienced less physical and mental quality of life improvement six months later. On the other hand, the women who were more likely to seek out information about their illness experienced greater physical quality of life improvement. The authors concluded that focusing on symptoms is a maladaptive approach to illness, but that information seeking may yield benefits to physical recovery.

Coping and Survival

Long-term survival is often used as an outcome measure of breast cancer treatment. Survival is relatively easy to define, but usually death from any cause is used and not only death caused by the breast cancer.

A multicentre study from Norway showed survival data for a follow-up of eight years for 515 cancer patients. The survival rate was lower for users of alternative medicine, 21%, compared to non-users, 35%. The authors concluded that use of alternative medicine may predict a shorter survival (Risberg, et al 2003).

Aim

The use of CAM has been associated with greater psychosocial distress and a poorer quality of life. Coping is defined as cognitive and behavioural ways to handle stress and perceived quality of life could be looked upon as an outcome of coping. The aim of the present study was to study the relation between coping, quality of life and survival in two samples of women with breast cancer, in anthroposophic and conventional care respectively. Another aim was to study the stability of ways of coping over time and whether it would be possible to predict quality of life and survival at a later time from coping at a specific time.

Research Questions

1. Are there any differences in perceived quality of life between women with different ways of coping at admission to the study and in comparison with Swedish women in general?
2. What are the relations between way of coping, cancer stage and time since diagnosis?
3. What are the relations between way of coping and perceived quality of life in women in anthroposophic care and conventional care over a five year period?
4. How stable are way of coping over a five year period in women in anthroposophic care and conventional care respectively?
5. Is it possible to predict quality of life after six months, one and five years from way of coping at admission to the study?
6. Are there any relations between way of coping at admission to the study and survival after one and five years?

The present study is part of a major clinical study of the outcome of anthroposophic medicine and care for women with breast cancer. Results have earlier been published (Arman et al, 2001, Carlsson et al 2001; 2004; 2005; 2006; Arman and Backman 2007).

Methods

Design and Sample

Data from a longitudinal study of the outcome of anthroposophic and conventional medicine and care for women with breast cancer were used. The women were followed for five years on six different data collection points. Data were collected (1) at admission to the study, (2) after 1 month, (3) after 3 months, (4) after 6 months, (5) after 1 year, and (6) after 5 years. In all 120 women took part in the main study, 60 who chose an anthroposophic hospital for treatment and 60 individually matched women from an oncology out-patient department who received conventional medical treatment. The inclusion criteria were age 75 years old or younger, living in the Stockholm-region, being able to communicate in Swedish, and being expected to live at least 6 months. Sixty women from the anthroposophic hospital were included from November 1995 to January 2000. During that time, 68 women who fulfilled the inclusion criteria were asked for participation and 60 agreed. Each of these women was individually matched with a woman who received conventional medical treatment. The women were followed for 5 years, which means that the data collection period started 1995 and ended 2005. The matching criteria were (1) stage of disease (advanced cancer or local limited cancer), (2) age (above 50 or below 50 years of age) (3) treatment during the last 3 months (radiotherapy/chemotherapy or no treatment), and (4) prognosis due to metastasis and the localization of the metastasis (favourable or unfavourable prognosis). The participants and the matching criteria are presented in table 1.

Table 1. The participants and the matching criteria

Sociodemographics	Women in Antroposophic care n=60	Women in conventional care n=60
Age	M=49.3 years, SD=9.7	M=49.1 years, SD=8.5
Living with partner	40	47
Having children	45	51
Professions		
Teachers	11	9
Salaried employees	15	23
Nurses	14	14
Journalists and artists	14	0
Other	3	8
Retired	3	5
Matching criteria		
Disease stage		
Advanced	42	42
Limited	18	18
Age		
>50 years	20	20
$\leq$ 50 years	40	40
Treatment 3 months prior to admission		
Treatment	41	41
No treatment	19	19
Prognosis		
Favourable	35	35
Non-favorable	25	25

The women were followed for five years. The women in both groups were treated according to a special regional care program for patients in the Stockholm/Gotland region. (Rutqvist et al, 1996). The women in anthroposophic care were additionally treated with a special care program at an anthroposophic hospital (Mean stay 14. 3 days; range 5-29 days). The anthroposophic therapies were individually composed and could be described as holistic care including natural products, Iscador (mistletoe extract), diet, art, rhythmic therapy, therapeutic massage, and hydrotherapy (Evans, 1992).

The Instruments

The Mental Adjustment to Cancer Scale

The MAC-scale consists of 40 items answered on 4-point scales. Example:" I feel that there is nothing I can do to help myself". Responses range from *(1) definitely does not apply to me* to *(4) definitely applies to me.* The MAC-scale contains five subscales: Fighting Spirit (FS), Helpless/Hopeless (HH), Anxious Preoccupation (AP), Fatalism (FA), and Avoidance (A) (Watson et al, 1988; Watson et al, 1999). In the present study the scales HH, AP, FA and A were combined to a variable representing passive and/or anxious behaviour (PAC) (Carlsson et al, 2005). The raw scores of the items were summarized, divided by the highest point in the scale and multiplied by 100. Thus, 100 represent the maximum use of each coping strategy.

The EORTC QLQ-C30

The EORTC QLQ-C30 consists of 30 items expressed in six functional scales (PF= physical functioning, RF= role functioning, EF= emotional functioning, CF= cognitive functioning, SF= social functioning, and QL= global quality of life), and nine symptom scales (FA= fatigue, NV= nausea and vomiting, PA= pain, DY= dyspnea, SL= sleep disturbance, AP=appetite loss, CO= constipation, DI= diarrhea, and FI= financial impact). The Swedish edition of version 1.0 of the instrument was used (Borghede et al, 1997). The scores of the functional scales are linearly transformed such that all scales range from 0 to 100, with a higher scale score representing a higher level of functioning. The symptoms scale items are also linearly transformed such that all scales/items range from 0 to 100. Higher sores represent a higher level of symptoms/problems (Borghede et al, 1997; Fayers et al, 1999). In the present study the six functional scales were used.

The Life Satisfaction Questionnaire (LSQ)

The LSQ consist of 34 items on 7-point scales. Examples : "How much have you been troubled by tiredness during the last week?". Responses range from *"1" very much* to "*7*", *not at all.* Scale point 7 represents the highest quality in all items. The 34 items are allocated to six different factors: physical symptoms (PS), sickness impact (SI), quality of daily activities (QDA), socioeconomic situation (SES), quality of family relation (QFA), and quality of close friend relationship (QFR). The raw scores of the items are summarized, divided by the highest point in the scale and multiplied by 100. Thus, 100 represent the maximum quality in each factor. The total quality of life-score is calculated in the same way. (Carlsson et al, 2002).

Procedure

The scales FS and PAC were dichotomized by the median. (Md= 72.6 for FS and Md= 47.9 for PAC). The 120 women were then categorized into four categories: low copers, which meant low in FS and low in PAC, high copers, high in FS and high in PAC, emotional copers, low in FS and high in PAC, and fighters, high in FS and low in PAC.

Data Analysis

Descriptive statistics, Chi-square, independent t-tests and analyses of variance (ANOVA) were used. SPSS version 14.0 was used for the statistical procedures.

Ethical Considerations

The main project, the study of the outcome of anthroposophic medicine, has been approved after ethical investigation by the Regional Research Ethics Committee at the Karolinska Institute, Stockholm, in 1995 and 2001.

Findings

Perceived Quality of Life in Women with Different Ways of Coping at Admission to the Study and a Comparison with Swedish Women in General

At admission to the study the women were categorised according to their way of coping. In table 2 the distribution of women in the different coping categories are presented.

Table 2. The distribution of women in different coping categories at admission to the study

Coping category	Women in Antroposophic care n=60	Women in conventional care n=60	n
Low copers	10	10	20
High copers	13	13	26
Emotional copers	24	16	40
Fighters	13	21	34

There where no significant differences between the groups women in anthroposophic care and women in conventional care regarding ways of coping (Chi-square = 3.482, DF=3, p=0.323

There were significant differences in assessed quality of life between the women called fighters compared to the women in the other groups. These differences are presented in tables 3 and 4 and figure 1. Most differences were found between fighters and the other ways of coping. This is also illustrated in figure 1.

Table 3. Means and Standard Deviations in quality of life at admission to the study for the women in the coping categories low copers, high copers, emotional copers, and fighters

	Sign	Low copers		High copers		Emotional copers		Fighters	
Scale	P	M	SD	M	SD	M	SD	M	SD
PF*	n.s.	60.2	30.4	71.5	24.8	66.5	26.2	78.8	24.6
RF	n.s	62.5	27.5	57.7	30.6	45.3	33.7	61.8	34.9
EF	0.000	66.7	19.9	65.4	26.0	46.9	19.7	74.5	22.0
CF	0.003	69.2	23.7	72.4	24.5	62.5	27.2	83.8	19.1
SF	0.002	60.8	32.6	61.5	30.1	45.8	29.3	75.0	24.4
QL	0.000	46.7	22.7	58.7	19.4	41.9	20.1	64.0	18.5
PS	0.000	81.5	12.6	81.4	11.6	77.0	14.2	90.5	10.6
SI	0.014	54.9	18.0	62.5	15.5	54.0	16.1	65.8	18.5
QDA	0.000	58.7	16.3	59.8	18.9	51.8	17.8	70.0	12.6
SES	0.000	65.8	14.7	72.2	16.1	56.9	16.3	79.2	8.5
QFA	0.037	74.6	16.1	71.4	17.0	72.1	19.6	82.1	11.6
QFR	0.004	75.3	11.6	76.7	14.0	71.9	13.4	82.6	10.5
QoLot	0.000	68.5	9.4	70.7	9.9	64.0	10.6	78.4	7.0

PF= physical functioning, RF= role functioning, EF= emotional functioning, CF= cognitive functioning, SF= social functioning, QL= global quality of life, PS= physical symptoms, SI= sickness impact, QDA= quality of daily activities, SES= socioeconomical situation, QFA= quality of family relation, QFR= quality of close friend relation, QoLtot= overall quality of life

Table 4. Significant differences in quality of life between women with different ways of coping

	Low	High	Emotional	Fighter
Low		QL	EF SF QLtot	CF QL PS SI QDA, SES QFR QLtot
High			EF SES,QLtot	PS SI QDA QFA QLtot
Emotional				EF CF SF QL PS SI QDA SES QFA QLtot

A comparison with a random sample of Swedish women in general aged 18-80 regarding perceived over all quality of life (M= 75.79, SD= 9.63) measured by the LSQ (Carlsson and Hamrin, 2002), showed that low copers assessed lower quality of life than Swedish women in general, (p= 0.003), high copers also assessed lower over all quality of life (p= 0.014), as did emotional copers (p= 0.000) but fighters assessed higher quality of life compared to Swedish women in general (p= 0.038).

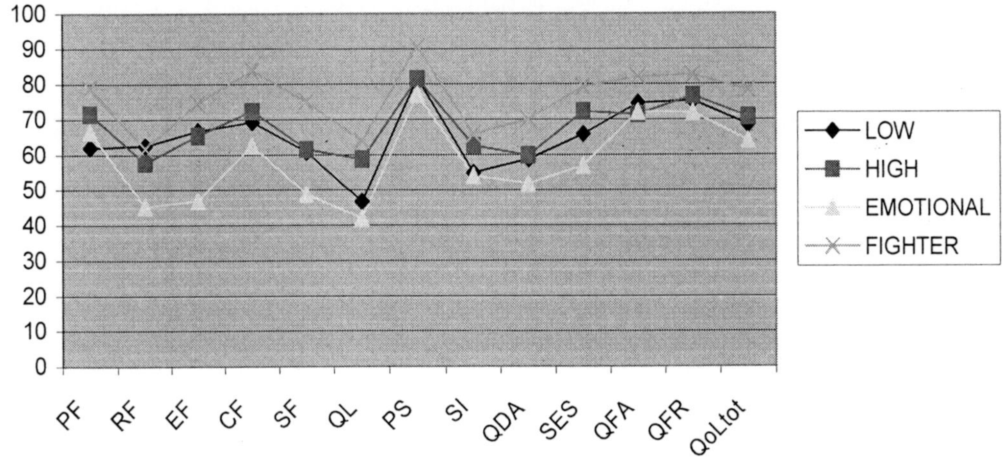

Figure 1. Perceived quality of life in women with different ways of coping at admission to the study.

The Relations between Way of Coping, Cancer Stage and Time Since Diagnosis

There were no significant differences between the women in the different coping categories regarding cancer stage or time since diagnoses at admission to the study. These data are presented in table 5.

Table 5. Cancer stage and time since diagnoses in women in the different coping categories at admission to the study

Coping	Limited cancer	Advanced cancer	Time since diagnosis
Low	7	13	M= 33.5 months, SD= 32.9
High	6	20	M= 36.1 months, SD= 34.8
Emotional	12	28	M= 39.3 months, SD= 51.4
Fighter	11	23	M= 29.1 months, SD= 39.0

The Relation between Way of Coping and Perceived Quality of Life in Women in Anthroposophic Care and Conventional Care over a Five Year Period

Between the first and the second data collection points the women were treated either at an anthroposophic hospital or at a conventional medical clinic. In the following text the groups are presented separately

The Women in Anthroposophic Care

In table 6 the relation between ways of coping and quality of life at every data collection points is presented. Over-all quality of life measured by the LSQ was chosen for the comparisons.

Table 6. The relation between ways of coping and over-all quality of life in the women treated in anthroposophic care. Means, Standard Deviations, F and p-values

Data collection	Low			High			Emotional			Fighter			F	p
	M	SD	N	M	SD	n	M	SD	n	M	SD	N		
I*	66.7	5.4	10	66.8	8.2	13	63.3	9.5	24	79.2	6.3	13	11.23	0.000
II	73.3	8.1	18	71.4	9.8	11	62.3	10.4	15	78.5	9.6	8	6.268	0.001
III	70.1	7.9	15	73.3	7.2	10	62.1	8.4	11	77.1	10.2	15	6.275	0.001
IV	73.1	10.6	14	71.3	8.9	16	69	6.8	8	77.6	10.8	10	1.407	0.253
V	75.4	8.5	20	71	11.5	8	70	7.8	9	85.8	8	4	3.362	0.029
VI	69.5	12.6	7	68.8	4.6	2	75.3		1	80.6	6.6	7	1.751	0.206

* I= admission, II= after 1 month, III= after 3 months, IV= after 6 months, V=after 1 year, VI= after 5 years.

The significant differences between the different ways of coping at the different data collection points are presented in table 7.

Table 7. Significant differences over time between women with different ways of coping in anthroposophic care

Category	Low	High	Emotional	Fighter
Low			III	I*; III; V
High			II; III	I; V
Emotional				I; II; III; V

* I= admission, II= after 1 month, III= after 3 months, IV= after 6 months, V=after 1 year, VI= after 5 years.

The Women in Conventional Care

In table 8 the relation between ways of coping and over-all quality of life in the women treated in conventional care over time is shown.

The significant differences between the different ways of coping at the different data collection points are presented in table 9.

Way of Coping over Time

In table 10 the number of women who had changed their way of coping compared to admission at the different data collection points during the 5-year data collection period in the two groups of women are presented.

There were changes over time in ways of coping in both groups. There was a significant difference between the groups after 6 months and after 5 years. More women in anthroposophic care had changed their way of coping compared to the women in conventional care.

A total of 88 women survived for 1 year and answered the MAC-scale. Among those there were 23 who rated their way of coping to be the same at all data collection points (data are not shown in any table). That means that about 26% of the women showed persistent coping and 74% changed their way of coping during one year. There was a significant difference between the groups (Chi-square= 7.729, DF= 1, p= 0.005). Five women out of 41 who got anthroposophic treatment showed persistent coping pattern throughout the year, which is about 12%. Of the women on conventional treatment, 18 out of 47 showed a persistent coping pattern, which is about 38%.

Of the 41 women who survived for 5 years and who answered the MAC-scale, 9 women rated their coping to be the same on all occasions. That means that about 22% of the women showed persistent coping and 78% changed their way of coping during five year. One woman out of 19 who got anthroposophic treatment showed persistent coping pattern throughout the years. Of the women in conventional treatment, 8 out of 22 showed a persistent coping pattern. Of the 9 women who assessed persistent way of coping, 6 were fighters, 2 low copers and 1 emotional coper.

Table 8. The relation between ways of coping and over-all quality of life in the women treated in conventional care. Means, Standard Deviations, F and p-values

Data collection	Low			High			Emotional			Fighter			F	p
	M	SD	N	M	SD	n	M	SD	n	M	SD	N		
I *	70.2	12.3	10	74.5	10.3	13	64.9	12.3	16	77.9	7.5	21	5.083	0.003
II	72	12.9	14	79.1	12.3	6	65.7	9.9	18	76.5	10	19	3.837	0.015
III	69.6	8.4	14	76.6	21.5	7	59.8	12	14	78.6	9.9	20	7.241	0.000
IV	71.7	12.2	12	82.8	12.2	6	63.6	9.3	17	77	9.2	18	7.329	0.000
V	68.6	11.8	10	68.3	7.5	5	59.2	9.8	12	78.8	10.6	19	8.906	0.000
VI	75.7	9.7	9	76.8	76.8	1	70.9	28.5	2	79.4	10.5	10	0.343	0.794

* I= admission, II= after 1 month, III= after 3 months, IV= after 6 months, V=after 1 year, VI= after 5 years.

Table 9. Significant differences over time between women with different ways of coping in conventional care

Category	Low	High	Emotional	Fighter
Low		IV	III; IV; V	III; V
High			I*; II; III; IV	
Emotional				I; II; III; IV; V

* I= admission, II= after 1 month, III= after 3 months, IV= after 6 months, V=after 1 year, VI= after 5 years.

Table 10. The number of women who had changed way of coping at the different data collection points compared to admission in the two groups of women

	Women in anthroposophic care			Women in conventional care				
	Changed	Unchanged	n	Changed	Unchanged	n	Chi-square	p
I-II*	24	29	53	21	37	58	0.946	0.218
I-III	24	27	51	23	32	55	0.294	0.364
I-IV	31	18	49	23	30	53	4.035	0.035
I-V	20	21	41	21	26	47	0.701	0.432
I-VI	14	5	19	7	15	22	7.152	0.009

*I = admission, II= after 1 month, III= after 3 months, IV= after 6 months, V= after 1 year, VI= after 5 years.

Prediction of Quality of Life after Six Months, One and Five Years from Way of Coping at Admission to the Study

In table 11 the perceived over all quality of life at 6 months, 1 year and 5 years for the women with different ways of coping at admission to the study in women in anthroposophic and conventional care respectively is presented.

For the women in anthroposophic care there were significant differences in assessed quality of life at 6 months (F= 4.681, p= 0.006) and after 1 year (F= 3.947, p= 0.015) between different ways of coping. The women in anthroposophic care who where categorised as fighters assessed significantly higher quality of life at 6 months than women categorised as high or emotional copers, and significantly higher quality of life than emotional copers after 1 year.

Way of Coping and Survival after 1 and 5 Years

In table 12 the relation between way of coping at admission to the study and survival after 1 year is presented.

There were no differences between women with different ways of coping at admission to the study concerning survival after 1 year.

In table 13 the relation between way of coping at admission to the study and survival after 5 years is presented.

Table 11. Overall quality of life after 6 months, 1 year and after 5 years in women with different ways of coping at admission to the study in women in anthroposophic and conventional care respectively

Coping category	6 months				1 year				5 years			
	A*		C**		A		C		A		C	
	M	SD	M	SD	M	SD	M	SD	M	SD	M	SD
Low	72.1	8.8	74.5	14.6	73.3	10.7	68.1	14.7	75.3	8.0	73.1	10.2
High	67.5	9.1	69.2	11.4	71.1	9.0	70.8	13.6	68.8	4.6	72.1	13.0
Emotional	71.1	7.1	67.8	10.3	71.3	6.9	65.3	14.4	76.0	12.1	88.4	3.8
Fighter	80.9	10.6	75.8	11.9	82.6	10.4	75.5	11.2	77.5	10.3	78.9	10.7
n	48		53		41		47		21		23	

*A = Women in anthroposophic care
** C= Women in conventional care.

Table 12. Coping at admission to the study and survival after 1 year in women in anthroposophic care and conventional care respectively

	Women in anthroposophic care			Women in conventional care		
Coping category	Still alive	deceased	n	Still alive	deceased	n
Low coper	9	1	10	8	2	10
High coper	9	4	13	9	4	13
Emotional coper	20	4	24	13	3	16
Fighter	10	3	13	20	1	21
Chi-square	1.811; DF=3			4.134; DF= 3		
P	0.631			0.247		

Table 13. Coping at admission of the study and survival after 5 year in women in anthroposophic care and conventional care respectively

	Women in anthroposophic care			Women in conventional care		
Coping category	Still alive	deceased	N	Still alive	deceased	n
Low coper	5	5	10	6	4	10
High coper	3	10	13	7	6	13
Emotional coper	13	11	24	5	11	16
Fighter	5	8	13	13	8	21
Chi-square	3.626; DF=3			3.855; DF=3		
P	0.305			0.278		

There were no differences between women with different ways of coping at admission to the study concerning survival after 5 years

Conclusion

The result showed that there were differences in perceived quality of life between women with different ways of coping at admission to the study. The women categorised as fighters assessed higher quality of life compared to the other women. The comparison with Swedish women in general showed that low copers, high copers and emotional copers assessed lower quality of life. The women called fighters, on the other hand, assessed significantly higher quality of life compared to Swedish women in general. There was no relation between cancer stage, time since diagnosis and way of coping. The women in anthroposophic care as well as the women in conventional care showed the same pattern over time, emotional copers assessed lower quality of life compared to fighters and high copers. Some of the women assessed the same way of coping at all data collection points, but most of them did not. More women in conventional care showed persistent coping compared to the women in anthroposophic care. For the women in anthroposophic care it was possible to predict that women who were categorised as fighters at admission to the study would score higher quality of life than women who were categorised as emotional copers after six months and after one year. But it was not possible to predict survival after one or five years from way of coping at admission to the study.

That the women categorised as fighters assessed higher quality of life compared to the other women is in agreement with other studies (Greer, 1991; Schnoll et al, 1998). According to Osoba et al (1998) a difference of 10 points on a 100- point scale could be considered a significant difference of clinical importance. That means that the differences in assessed quality of life between the women categorised as fighters and the other women in the present study, are of importance. The result also showed that the women categorised as fighters assessed higher quality of life compared to Swedish women in general. This is an interesting finding since it means that it is possible to live with breast cancer and still have a high quality of life. Another important result of the present study was that ways of coping could change over time and more so in the women treated in anthroposophic care. In both groups there were women who changed their way of coping. The result of the present study is in agreement with the assumption that coping is a process or a state that varies over time rather than a trait, since only about 20-25% of the women assessed the same coping over time. Most women changed their way of coping and that was more obvious among the women who were treated within anthroposophic care. Maybe the individually composed anthroposophic therapies helped the women to change their coping. This is only a suggestion and the explanation is beyond the scope of the present paper. Manuel et al (2007) concluded that positive cognitive restructuring was the most helpful way to cope with concerns about the future, and Ransom et al (2005) showed that information seeking about the illness could be positive for physical quality of life. But to deal with anger and depression, social support seemed to be most helpful (Manuel et al. 2007). Thus, research is needed to understand how coping could be strengthened or changed in order to attain optimal quality of life in dealing with different problems in different phases of life.

There was no relation between ways of coping, cancer stage, time since diagnosis, or survival in any of the two groups of women. Coping is a psychological variable and the present study gave no evidence for any association between coping and the course of cancer. This result is in agreement with the result of a study by Godwin et al (2005), who concluded that evidence of how psychosocial status and health-related quality of life is associated with breast cancer outcome is weak and inconsistent.

Twenty six (43%) of the women in anthroposophic care and 31 (52%) in conventional care survived the five year data collection period (see table 13). This difference is not statistically significant ($p= 0.132$) but the tendency is in agreement with the result of the study by Risberg et al (2003). Studies have shown that women who choose alternative and complementary medicine tend to have more psychological problems and to adopt a more depressive coping strategy (Moschen et al 2001; Risberg, 2003; Cassileth and Deng, 2004) In the present study there was a significant difference in over all quality of life between the women in anthroposophic care and the women in conventional care at admission to the study. ($M(A)= 68.08$, $SD= 9.9$, $M(C)= 72.42$, $SD= 11.39$, $p= 0.028$).

Study Limitations and Strength

There are limitations of the study that should be considered. The design of the study is one. The women were not randomised to the two treatment groups, anthroposophic care and conventional care. The women were matched regarding age, stage of disease, treatment during the 3 months before admission to the study, and prognosis. The women who choose anthroposophic care was the starting point and the other group was created according to the matching criteria. But the differences between the groups were in agreement with what have been found in other studies (Moschen et al 2001; Risberg, 2003; Cassileth and Deng, 2004). Thus it might be suggested that the women in the present study were representative of women in anthroposophic care and conventional care respectively.

Another limitation is the sample size. One hundred and twenty women were included, but after five years there were only 41 women left who had answered the questionnaires. That means there could be a risk of Type II error.

The use of the MAC-scale was not according to the manual and that might be seen as a limitation. To categorise women into the four categories low copers, high copers, emotional copers and fighters could be questioned, but it seemed logical from the theoretical assumptions about coping to be either problem focused or emotion focused. (Lazarus and Folkman, 1984; Lazarus, 1993, Lindqvist et al, 2000).

The strength of the study is that the instruments used to measure quality of life/ life satisfaction and coping have been tested for reliability and validity and show acceptable psychometric properties. (Fayers et al 1999; Nordin et al, 1999; Carlsson et al, 2002).

The conclusion of the study was that there is an obvious relation between way of coping and the perceived quality of life. The women categorised as fighters assessed significantly higher quality of life than the other women and also higher than Swedish women in general. Most women changed their ways of coping over the five year period and that was more obvious for the women who were treated within anthroposophic care. There was no relation found between ways of coping and cancer stage, time since diagnosis, or survival.

Acknowledgments

The study was supported by the Swedish Council of Planning and Co-ordination of Research (No: 950204:6), the Swedish Cancer Society (No: 3684-B95-01XAB; 3684-B96-02XBB; No 3684-B97-03XAA), the Gyllenberg Foundation, Finland and the Agape Foundation, Sweden. Receiver of grants: Elisabeth Hamrin.

References

Anderson RT, Aaronson NK, Wilkin D. Critical review of the international assessments of health-related quality of life. *Qual. Life Res.* 1993; 2: 369-395.

Arman M, Backman M. A longitudinal study on women's experiences of life with breast cancer in anthroposophical (complementary) and conventional care. *European Journal of Cancer Care,* 2007; 16(5):444-450

Arman M, Rhensfeldt A, Carlsson M, Hamrin E. Indications of change in life perspective among women with breast cancer admitted to complementary care. *European Journal of Cancer Care,* 2001; 10: 192-200.

Borghede G, Karlsson J, Sullivan M. Quality of life in patients with prostate cancer. Results from a Swedish population study. *J. Uro.* 1997; 158:1477-85.

Carlsson M, Arman M, Backman M, Hamrin E. Perceived quality of life and coping for Swedish women with breast cancer who choose complementary medicine. *Cancer Nursing,* 2001; 24 (5): 395- 401.

Carlsson M, Hamrin E. Evaluation of the life satisfaction questionnaire (LSQ) using structural modelling (SEM). *Qual. Life Res.* 2002; 11: 415-25.

Carlsson M, Hamrin E. The Life Satisfaction Questionnaire (LSQ). Manual. Uppsala: Department of Public Health and Caring Sciences, Uppsala University and Linköping: Department of Medicine and Care, University of Linköping, 2002

Carlsson M, Arman M, Backman M, Flatters U, Hatschek T, Hamrin E. Evaluation of quality of life/life satisfaction in women with breast cancer in complementary and conventional care *Acta Oncol.* 2004; 43 (1):27-34.

Carlsson M, Arman M, Backman M, Hamrin E. Coping in women with breast cancer in complementary and conventional care over 5 years, measured by the Mental Adjustment to Cancer scale *JACM.* 2005; 11(3): 441-447.

Carlsson M, Arman M, Backman M, Flatters U, Hatschek T, Hamrin E. A five-year follow-up of quality of life in women with breast cancer in anthroposophic and conventional care. *Evid Based Complement and Alternat Med,* 2006 ; 3(4):523-531.

Cassileth BR, Schraub S, Robinson E, Vickers A. Alternative Medicine use world wide, *Cancer.* 2001; 91:1390-3.

Cassileth BR, Deng G. Complementary and alternative therapies for cancer. *Oncologist.* 2004; 9:80-9.

Evans M, Rodger I. Anthroposophical Medicine: Healing for Body, Soul and Spirit. London: Thorsons, 1992.

Fayers P, Aaronsin N, Bjordal K, Curran D, Groenvold M. Scoring manual. Brussels: EORTC Quality of Life Study Group; 1999. (http://www.eortc.be/home/qol/manuals.htm).

Goldstein MS, Brown ER, Ballard-Barbash R, Morgenstern H, BastaniR, Lee J et al. The use of complementary and alternative medicine among Californian adults with and without cancer. *Evid. Based Complement. Alternat. Med.* 2005; 2: 557-65.

Goodwin PJ, Ennis M, Bordeleau LJ, Pritchard KI, Trudeau ME, Koo J, Hood N. Helath-related quality of life and psychosocial status in breast cancer prognosis: analysis of multiple variables. *J. Clin. Oncology.* 2005 20; 23(6): 1335-6.

Greer S. Psychological responses to cancer and survival *Psychol. Med,* 1991; 21:43-9.

LaFortune Fredette S. breast cancer survivors: Concerns and coping. *Cancer Nursing,* 1995; 18(1): 35-46.

Lauver DR, Connolly-Nelsson K, Vang P. Stressors and coping strategies among female cancer survivors after treatment. *Cancer Nursing.* 2007; 30(2):101-111.

Lazarus R. Coping theory and research: Past, Present and Future. *Psychosom. Med.* 1993; 55:234-247.

Lazarus RS, Folkman S. *Stress, Appraisal and Coping.* New York: Springer, 1984

Lehto US, Ojanen M, Dyba T, Aromaa A, Kellokumpu-Lehtinen P. Baseline psychosocial predictors of survival in localised breast cancer, *Br. J. Cancer.* 1006 8; 94 (9): 1245-52.

Lindqvist R, Carlsson M, Sjödén PO. Coping strategies and styles assessed by the Jalowiec Coping Scale in a random sample of the Swedish population. *Scand. J. Caring. Sci.* 2000;14:147-154.

Manuel JC, Burwell SR, Crawford SL, Lawrence RH, Farmer DF, Hege A, Phillips K, Avis NE. Younger women's perception of coping with breast cancer. *Cancer Nursing.* 2007; 30(2):85-94.

Moschen R, Kemmler G, Schweigkofler H, Holzner B, Dunser M, Richter R, Fleischhacker WW, Sperner-Unterweger B. Use of alternative/complementary therapy in breast cancer patients – a psychological perspective. *Supportive Care in Cancer,* 2001, 9(4):267-274.

Nordin K. Psychological responses to gastrointestinal cancer (dissertation) Uppsala: Acta Universitatis Upsaliensis. *Comprehensive Summaries of Uppsala Dissertations from Faculty of Medicine,* No,779, 1998

Nordin K, Berglund G, Terje I, Glimelius B. The Mental Adjustment to Cancer Scale. A psychometric analysis and the concept of coping. *Psychooncology,* 1999;8:250-259.

Osoba D, Rodrigues G, Myles J, Zee B, Pater, J. Interpreting the significance of changes in health-related quality of life scores. *J. Clinical. Oncology,* 1998; 16 (1): 139-144.

Ransom S, Jacobsen PB, Schmidt JE, Andrykowski MA. Relationship of problem-focused coping strategies to changes in quality of life follwoing treatment for early stage breast cancer. *J. Pain Symptom Manage,* 2005 Sep;30(3):243-53.

Risberg T, Jacobsen BK. The association between mental distress and the use of alternative medicine among cancer patients in North Norway. *Qual Life Res.* 2003; 12(5):539-44.

Risberg T Kolstad A, Cassileth BR. Use of alternative medicine among Norwegian cancer patients associated with mental distress – a follow up study. *Acta Oncol.* 2002; 41(7-8):646-51

Risberg T Vickers A, Bremnes RM Wist EA Kaasa S, Cassileth BR. Does use of alternative medicine predict survival from cancer? *Eur. J. Cancer.* 2003 Jul;39(11): 1642

Rutqvist LE, Fornander T, Fernstedt R, Wilking N, Bäckdahl M, Skoog L et al. Bröstcancer. Diagnostik, behandling och uppföljning i Stockholm-Gotland regionen. Vårdprogram. (Breast cancer. Diagnostics, Treatment and Follow-up in the Stockholm-Gotland Region. Care Program, in Swedish). Stockholm: Onkologiskt Centrum Stockholm- Gotland, 1996.

Schnoll RA, Harlow LL, Brandt U, Stohlbach LL. Using two factor structure of the Mental Adjustment to Cancer (MAC) Scale for assessing adaptation to breast cancer. *Psychooncology.* 1998;7:424-435.

Smith K, Avis N, Assman S. Distinguishing between quality of life and health status in quality of life research: A meta-analysis. *Qual. Life Res.* 1999; 8:447-459.

Watson M, Greer S, Young J, Inayat Q, Burgess C, Robertson B. Development of a questionnaire measure adjustment to cancer: the MAC scale. *Psychology and Medicine.* 1988; 18:203-209.

Watson M, Haviland JS, Greer S, Davidson J; Bliss JM. Influence of psychological response on survival in breast cancer: a population-based cohort study. *Lancet.* 1999; 354: 1331-36.

In: Coping with Cancer
Editor: Léa K. Jacobs, pp. 127-140

ISBN: 978-1-60456-213-2

Chapter VI

Cancer as a Family Affair: How the Illness Influences Family Life - a Nursing Science Perspective

Katharina Lex
Unversität Witten/Herdecke

Abstract

In Germany, every Year some 425,000 people are newly diagnosed with cancer. About 217,000 people of them will die [1]. Not only is the patient suddenly confronted with enormous stress. As the majority of the German population is surrounded by "relevant other people"- family, friends, colleagues, neighbours etc.- many more people than those having been diagnosed suffer from the cancer [2, 3, 4, 5]. In this chapter I shall give an overview over the areas of family life which might be affected by the illness. After an introduction I shall comment on the new family concept and discuss effects on partnerships, children and communication patterns within families. I shall then examine family coping strategies and responsibilities for nurses. In my conclusion I aim to show some of the challenges for the nursing profession working with cancer patients.

Introduction

In Germany, every Year some 425 000 people are newly diagnosed with cancer. About 217 000 of them will die [1]. Not only the patient is suddenly confronted with enormous stress. As the majority of the German population is surrounded by "relevant other people" (family, friends, collegues, neighbours etc.) many more people than those having been diagnosed suffer from the cancer [2, 3, 4, 5]. In recent years, cancer has more and more changed from an acute illness to a chronic disease. These changes occured through more efficient diagnoses and therapeutic possibilities [6].

Cancer patients and their families are being increasingly confronted with the following problems:

- The complexity of medical and nursing care can be confusing as differnet medical disciplines tend to be involved in the care and therapy of cancer patients [7]. This often makes it often difficult to keep close contact to the main health care providers.
- Throughout the course of the disease several hospitalizations might be necessary [7].
- Treatment costs may be high because of the use of highly developed treatment options [7].
- The onset of cancer can be slow and is often invisible [8].
- Cancer patients and their families may have to face economic hardship that may hit them quite suddenly [9, 10, 7, 11].
- Sometimes the aim of medical treatment changes from a "cure perspective" to a palliative care perspective. These changes may intensify feelings of anxiety and worry in the family because the patient will not survive the disease [7].

Apart from being suddenly confronted with a potential life threatening illness, one of the main challenges lies in the acceptance of new roles and the reorganization of daily life according to the demands of the disease [11]. Because patients have longer life expectancies, the periods in which one or several family members care for the patient, increase [12]. Due to demographic developments, nearly everybody nowadays has already been or will be a career in the future [13]. Before most family caregivers start to nurse a patient at home they tend not to be aware of and are therefore not well prepared, for the changes that might occur in their daily lives [14]. Nearly all ages are caring in family settings. The age spectrum starts with so called "young carers" (children who nurse their parents or grandparents). At the other end even very old people take over family nursing duties [13]. Carers within a marital relationship describe the changes they experience as shifting from "spouse" to "nurse" [14]. The identity of families is formed by traditions over generations and by shared plans for the future [15]. A potential life threatening illness like cancer often shatters these shared perspectives for the future [15]. Although the health care system becomes slowly aware of families and homes being a central place for nursing care, there still is an interesting discrepancy between the changes in family structures and shifting perceptions of families and the relevant nursing science research. My thesis is, that there is too little research in Germany about cancer in the family. The research results on the subject tend to be outdated, because the image of the family used in research is the classical family model that no longer is the only or even the most important model in modern families, and ultimately the families that are affected do not get the attention and help from nursing scientists they deserve and need. Research needs to focus on the specific situation in Germany taking its particular medical, nursing, social and family traditions into account. Still, there is a body of relevant research results that focus particularly on the needs of cancer patients, who are cared for at home and their families, partners and children. Although many families are willing to take on the amount of caring needed for a member that has been diagnosed with cancer, the strain of caring for an ill family member over a long period of time can lead to crises within these families [4]. These crises may prevent families from being able to nurse and care for the patient properly. Being not able to care for the patient may lead to the caring family member getting ill him- or herself [3, 14]. Other problems associated with family care are:

- Being inadequately prepared for the demands of care [14].
- Having to deal with possible side-effects of the treatment, for example-alopecia, nausea, emesis, and fatigue [10].
- Keeping the patient comfortable, especially if the patient is going to die from the cancer [7].
- Managing technical and nursing equipment, for example syringe drivers [7].
- Reporting adequately and quickly to the formal health care system if changes in the patients condition occur [7].
- Managing activities and responsibilities the patient had before falling ill [7].
- Managing difficult symptoms [7].
- Lacking time for oneself [14].
- Experiencing insufficient help from the formal healthcare system [14].

Due to the many challenges they have to face family caregivers may feel guilty and overwhelmed for example in situations where they cannot finish tasks they are doing [14]. Many carers experience feelings of strain, hardship and lack of control over demands, time and people [14]. Yet in spite of the enormous challenges of family care and the risk of crises some positive aspects associated with nursing a family member are mentioned in the literature:

- Greater emotional closeness with the patient [14].
- Satisfaction of giving care [14].
- Chance to return a favour to another person [14].

The nursing care a patient may need can differ considerably. The amount of caring depends on the following factors:

- Age of the patient [7].
- Disability and physical dependence of the patient [7].
- Relationship with the patient [7].
- Professional, social and family roles of the patient [7].
- Living conditions [7].
- Phase within the life circle of patient and carer [7].
- Experience and health of the main carer [7].
- Number of co-morbide conditions [7].
- Psychological condition [7].
- Cultural settings and traditions [7].
- Phase of the illness [7].
- Phase of the treatment [7].

Patient groups who receive relatively little support from their families tend to be female cancer patients, young cancer patients and long term cancer patients [16].The nursing care that is taken on by family members can vary widely. It depends not only on the degree of dependencies due to the illness but also on the relationships within the family. Relatives who take over activities from ill family members often do not describe their activities as "nursing" but as trying to live daily life under different circumstances [17]. Prolonged phases of illness can result in the deterioration of the emotional and physical family resources [18] and sometimes even the health of the main familial carer [14].

To be able to provide good care, carers need information and instructions in these fields:

- Diagnosis of the patient [13].
- Causes, significance, prevention and management of different symptoms [13].
- Nursing techniques [13].
- Realistic prognosis [13].
- Adequate reactions to sudden changes [13].
- Help in emergency situations [13].

Areas of family life that might be affected by the diagnosis include:

- Well-being of the children [8].
- Marital relationships [8].
- Communication within the family [19].
- Roles within the family [19].

The Concept "Family"

In western countries, an ideal of the "classical family" prevailed. According to this ideal, a family consisted of grandparents (married couples), parents (married couples), and a few children. This concept has changed dramatically in the recent past. Some nursing scientists claim now, that "family" consists of those persons that the person who is questioned says they are family, regardless of the persons mentioned being related to each other [20]. Because of this transformation of the classical family ideal nursing scientists use a model for families that is more realistic in the modern world [20]. Step by step the German nursing profession also gained greater awareness of families being one of the main contexts for nursing care, however one might define what the family is. The well - being of families does not only influence the functioning of families as a whole, but affects the well - being of each family member [3, 21]. It is known, that longer periods of illness can lead to a decline of the physical and psychological resources of a family [18]. Structurally and emotionally healthy families can usually take on new challenges, roles and forms of communication quite easily [22]. But even these "healthy families" can break down under the burden of having to live under an unpredictable period of time with a member that has been diagnosed with a potentially life threatening illness [22]. Apart from taking on nursing tasks the most important every day challenges for a family are dealing with the uncertainties of the illness [23], that are linked to the future of the family [24], then with the potential damages in the family's life cycle [24] and finally with shifts in the family structure [24]. Families that experience cancer are very concerned with firstly providing good care for the ill family member, secondly being united and supporting each other, and thirdly establishing and maintaining good relationships between the family and the professional care - giver [25].

Influences on the Partnership

Whereas there are some studies looking at the affects of the disease on communication and denial, anxieties and fears within a partnership research focussing on the effects of cancer on partnerships appears to concentrate on one aspect, the impact of cancer on the sexuality of the patient and the partner.

Not surprisingly, a study has shown that the spouse's anxiety increases when the other spouse tries to deny the situation [5]. Another study has pointed to the problem that many patients do not talk with their partner about sexual difficulties [26]. The patient does not want to burden their partner even more and the healthy partner wants to protect the ill partner [26]. Sexual difficulties often occur even before the diagnostic investigations have been completed [27]. Unspecific symptoms that often go along with a cancer diagnosis, for example pathologic bleedings, weight loss or pains can change persons self - image dramatically. That is why these symptoms may have a large influence on the sexuality of the patient [27]. The loss or the reduction of sexual sensations can have a major impact on the quality of life, self-esteem and satisfaction with the present living conditions of patient and his or her partner [26]. Younger patients suffer stronger from sexual difficulties than older patients [26]. The following factors have the potential to worsen sexual difficulties:

- Being unmarried [26].
- Having sexual activities with frequently changing partners [26].
- Having experienced sexual difficulties in the past [26].
- Having suffered the experience of sexual violence [26].

In general the reasons for sexual problems after receiving a cancer diagnosis can be put into one of these two groups:

- Physical reasons, for example discomfort or pain caused by cancers affecting the central nervous system (transverse lesion), invasive injuries surgery like a mastectomy, pains after operations, infertility after a hysterectomy [26].
- Psycho - social reasons,for example being upset about therapeutic interventions or about the illness itself, potential existing conflicts in the partnership getting worse because of the illness, false ideas about cancer, for example the worry to transmit cancer to the partner [26].

Influences on Children

According to recent statistics between 5% and 15% of all children younger than eighteen will be affected by one parent getting seriously physically ill [8]. About one person in three being diagnosed with cancer has, when the diagnosis is made, children who live at home [24]. It is estimated, that every year about 150 000 children in Germany are newly affected by their mothers or fathers being diagnosed with cancer [28]. For children it is often very difficult to come to terms with the new/changed family situation. There are estimates suggesting that about 50% of the affected children develop symptoms of the illness themselves if they do not receive professional help prophylactically. Other typical features can be behavioural difficulties, bad marks at school and social isolation [28]. For these children the risk of developing psychological illnesses later in life is twice as high as for "normal" children [28]. From several studies it is known, that parents tend to underestimate or not to realize any of the challenges their children have to face through their parents illness [10]. Astonishingly the coping mechanisms children use do not depend on the stage of their parents' illness but only on how the family as a whole deals with the illness [28]. Depending on the state of their cognitive development, children have different ideas about illness aetiologies of cancer and death. Younger children need visible signs, for example fever or lying in bed, to recognize that somebody is ill [7]. For very small children it is important, that the main person who is responsible for the child recognizes the child's needs quickly and reacts adequately to them [24]. Apart from that a positive and supporting presence of the caring adult is important [24].

Young children are often concerned with the following questions:

- Am I to blame for the illness [24]?
- Can I catch cancer myself [24]?
- Who will be looking after me [24]?

For young children it is necessary to spend a lot of time with their parents [24]. The changed daily routines should be adapted in spite of the parental disease to the needs of the children [24]. Information on the illness should be given adequately. This could be done, for example, through reading children's books together on the subject [24]. School aged children are often concerned with the following issues:

- Will the ill person die [24]?
- If, so will I have to go to a children's home [24]?
- What is going to happen if other important people like the other parent or the
- godparent get cancer as well [24]?
- Will we have less money [24]?
- Who will be looking after me if the parent is gone [24]?
- Can I influence the illness somehow [24]?

If the ill parent can not be with the child for longer periods of time, for example, because of protracted stays in a hospital, it might be helpful to keep contact through regular telephone calls or through pictures or text messages [24]. Talking about the illness should be made easy for the children [24]. If children feel encouraged to speak about their feelings and fears, the coping process might be easier for them [24]. Seeing friends is important for children of the age between 7 and 12 years [24]. Positive events, for example outings, can help children to come to terms with the changed family situation [24]. Adolescents tend to reflect on the aetiology of cancer and can be concerned with the risks of inheriting the disease themselves [8]. Even before parents have told their children about the cancer, many children suspect that "something is seriously wrong" [29]. These suspicions are drawn from observations on developments within the family, from the interpretation of their parents′ moods and from analyzing their parent's visits to medical facilities [29]. Most children develop, especially if they do not know precisely what is happening with their parents, a guilty conscience [30]. They may think, for example that the parent fell ill, because they misbehaved [30]. Many children connect the term "cancer" with death, although "only" about half of the people initially diagnosed with cancer will die from the disease [29, 1]. It is impossible, to protect a child from all the worries associated with the parental disease [7]. If children show one or more of these symptoms, they might need help:

- Withdrawal [24].
- Difficulties at school [24].
- Worries [24].
- Irritability [24].
- Bed wetting [24].
- Eating disorders [24].
- Frequent accidents [24].
- Risk - seeking behaviour [24].

There are several risk factors that increase the probability for children to develop psychological difficulties that are caused by their parent's diseases:

- Superficial family communication [28].
- Smouldering family conflicts [28].
- Social or emotional isolation of the family [28].
- Lack of support during important events for a child like the first day at school, a change of school, moves in the time of the parents' illness [28].
- Single parents [28].
- When mothers fall ill whose children are younger than eleven years old [28].
- When fathers fall ill of adolescent daughters [28].

Research has shown, that these are the main reasons, why parents should talk to their children about the parental cancer:

- Children's fantasies are often worse than the reality of the disease [8].
- Children might get wrong information from other people [8].

- Children might feel unimportant and excluded if they are not adequately informed on important events within the family [8].
- Parents do not have to waste energy for keeping the illness secret from the
- children [8].
- Even very sad realities are easier to live with than fear and uncertainty [8].

The better the information and preparation of children according to their age, their knowledge and their developmental state the better children will be able to cope [28, 10]. That is why it is recommended, that parents talk to their children about being ill [30]. Patients get in fact their main support for coping with their illness through their spouse and their children [31. A bad parent – child relationship during this crucial event of cancer in the family can lead to psychological disorders once the child has grown up [17]. It is recommended to wait and see when and how a child asks questions. It has been shown that the way patients are told about their disease has an impact on how well they manage to inform their children on the subject. To increase the probability that children become familiar with the parental disease it is necessary, that parents receive sufficient information about important aspects of their cancer. That will enable them to understand what is happening with them [32]. Parents need knowledge on the following questions to be able to prepare their children adequately for the new situation:

- How do children of a certain age deal with illness? Children's books on the
- subject cancer can be helpful in this situation [30].
- How do I know, that my child needs help [33]?
- What can I do if other children do not want to come into my house to visit my child [33]?
- What can I do if children do not want to share their anxieties with their parents [33]?
- How can I create opportunities for children to exchange their views on their
- parent's cancer with other children [30]?

Cancer can be the cause for communication within families to become more superficial. This kind of superficial communication can be used to cover up negative feelings like anxiety and stress [9]. Not only communication between partners can get difficult because of the illness, communication with children too might get more difficult. As some parents want to protect their children from fear and anxiety they do not tell their children about their mother or father been diagnosed with cancer [30, 28]. Open communication about the cancer and knowledge of possible outcomes of the disease may, however may lead to a reduction of anxiety in children [28].

Adolescents would like to have answers to the following questions:

- How serious is the disease [34]?
- What are possible side effects of the treatment [34]?
- Do alternative treatment options exist [34]?
- What possibilities are there to support the parents [34]?
- What are appropriate reactions, if the ill parent behaves strange [34]?

Adolescents find it important, to live a normal every day life in spite of a parent being ill. Meeting friends for example, matters [34]. Not surprisingly, the emotional difficulties of adolescents can get worse as soon as the tumour reoccurs [34]. The cancers reoccurrence may remind the adolescents that it is possible, that the parent will die from the cancer [34].

Family Coping Strategies

Coping with cancer is not only an important challenge for the patient, but also for the family, the colegues and neighbours who have to deal with the new situation [22]. Coping with cancer can be difficult because of the following reasons:

- Uncertainty about the aetiology of the disease [17].
- Lack of the preparedness of patient and surrounding family for what they might have to face in the future [36].
- Uncertainty about the duration of the care [14].
- Little scope to deal freely and independently with the disease and the treatment [36].
- The worst case scenario of a terminal prognossis [17].
- Anxiety about changes in the physical apearance of the patient, for example through operations or other medical treatment [17].

Considerable psycho-social burdens for thr patient and his family can occur depending on the phase of the illness, the expected prognosis and possible disabilities caused by the illness or the treatment [22]. Strong families with adequate resources including good socioemotional and economic support systems tend to be able to cope quite well [25]. Research has shown that skills, hope, optimism, humor and plans for the future are in fact helpful strategies for the patient and the family [25, 5]. One of the most powerfull factors to for coping well is being surrounded by other people [24]. Some other succesfull coping strategies include:

- Keeping up family unity [25].
- Working on a professional nurse-family relationship [25].

Hope seems to be an important coping strategie [9, 37]. Hope is not always aimed at the patient being cured from the disease [19]. Hope can also mean, that the patient gets the best possible care available and that suffering can be reduced [19]. Equally important are the feeling of remaining positive and the belief that one can bear the responsibility one has taken over through caring [14]. If there is anoften tacit agreement in the family on not to address the illness, this behaviour may lead to a “wall” of unaddressed emotions within the family [19]. If the patient does not feel able to talk about the illness, family or friends might feel completely excluded from the coping process [19]. This feeling can be very difficult to bear [19]. If the patient manages to live with the reality of the illness, partners, children and collegues will also learn to live with the situation [8]. As time goes by, families usually learn how to come to terms with the changed situation [37]. Research has demonstrated, that families take about one year to get used to the new situation [25].

Responsibilities for Nurses

Patients and families expect from the nurse to receive information on and help with nursing care, medication management, symptom assessment and communication with the formal health care team [11]. One task for the involved nurse is to clarify the patients and the family's needs and wishes [11]. An appropriate assessment is essential in order to allow meaningful interventions for the affected families [11]. As it is often a difficult task to judge children's reactions and needs for medical and nursing information, many families might find it less stressful, if they were offered help from medical professionals with fulfilling this task [28]. Frequently nurses notice, through their close contact with the families, which resources the family has. Through this knowledge, nurses are able to help the family to be "expert" on the nursing and care demands of their ill family members [38]. Nurses and other health care providers need to be aware of and prepared for strong ethnic racial and religious influences on perceptions of health and illness and the role of the family [39]. Helpful for family coping strategies might be if the nurse in charge works with the affected family works on the following tasks:

- Help family members to reorganize the family for continued care [25].
- Serve as an expert on illness information and management [25].
- Help families to see the impact of nursing care on the family and especially on the family members who are in charge of the care [25].
- Help families to solve problems accociated with the illness on their own [25].

The following questions can help nurses to discover the ressources and strengths of affected families:

- What parts of life changed through the illness [22]?
- What is the greatest problem for the family at this moment [19]?
- Who of the family members is having the worst time [19]?
- Who in the family talks about changes [22]?
- Which anxieties, whishes and hopes does the family have [22]?
- How did the family come to terms with difficoult situations in the past [22, 19]?
- Which ressources has the the patient and the partner to cope with this difficult situation [22, 19]?
- Who is most helpfull when dealing with the disease [22, 19]?
- Which kind of help does the family need [22]?
- What does the family expect from their future [22]?
- Doe the patient and the family talk about death [22, 19]?

Nurses and other health care professionals should be aware, that the information and support demands of caring family members vary widely [7].

Conclusion

So far, there is only relatively little nursing research in German dealing with the subject of caring for cancer patients in the family [40, 6]. There are no studies analyzing the particular German situation from a nursing science perspective. Considering the demographic developments it is surprising that nobody has done research in the German context exploring new concepts for helping families who have to live with chronic illness [3, 23]. Longitudinal studies on the subject, set in Germany, do not exist. The absence of this kind of studies is regrettable as there is a lack of information on long - term effects of cancer on affected families [7, 11]. Professional health care providers do not try hard enough to prepare families for the care process [25]. It seems as if professionals do not listen to the concerns families have when coping with the changes in daily family live [25]. Families need health care providers who are able to:

- Teach families on how to provide special nursing and medical care [25].
- Give family members information on the disease [25].
- Help to understand medical treatment options [25].
- Offer social and emotional support in times of crises [25].

None of the analysed studies focus on the situation of patients and families who have a great deal of problems apart from having to deal with a potentially life threatening illness [41]. These are, for example, families who already have to care for a family member in need, families in which several small children live, or families who do not have any financial or managerical resources [41]. So far, very little research has been done on coping with cancer set in "non - classical families" [41]. These families might be, for example, homosexual partnerships with children, single – parent families, families with a "migrational background" or patchwork families [41]. Another challenge leis in the juridical conditions in Germany. For a partner or friend who is not a blood relation or marital spouse, it is rather difficult to be included in the decision making process concerning the patient. The German system is very focused on the classical concept of families.

What makes the situation particularly difficult is the fact that nursing in Germany tends to be a very traditional profession which has difficulties with new challenges [42]. It will take presumably some time until it will be routine, for example, for homosexual partners of cancer patients to get involved into therapeutic and care decisions in the same way as partners in heterosexual partnerships. In the development of concepts that would help to establish a state of the art family nursing lies an enormous chance for the German nursing science profession. Additionally, better coordination and communication between the different health care providers should be encouraged [16]. For "bed side nursing" in Germany it will be important that the awareness of cancer as a family affair spreads. In daily life it might be helpful if nurses could cooperate more intensively with the people, who are the most important ones for the patient.

References

[1] http://www.destatis.de/basis/d/gesu/gesutab19.php (downloaded 9.6.2007)

[2] Woods, N., Lewis, F., Ellison, E. (1989). Living with cancer. Family experiences.*Cancer Nursing,* 12 (1), 28–33

[3] Controneo, M.; Zimmer, M.; Zegelin - Abt, A. (1999). Vorschläge für das Gesundheitssystem der Zukunft: Familienorientierte Primary *Health Care. Pflege,* 12, 163–171

[4] Schnepp, W. (2002). *Angehörige pflegen.* Hans Huber Verlag Bern

[5] Ben-Zur, H., Ora, G. , Lev, S. (2001). Coping With Breast Cancer: Patient, Spouse, and Dyad Models. *Psychosomatic Medicine,* 63, 32-39

[6] Lex, K. (2005). Krebs –was bedeutet das für die Familie? Gespräche nicht ins Stocken geraten lassen. *Pflegezeitschrift,* 2, 97-99

[7] Given, B.; Given, Ch.; Kozachik, S. (2001). Family Support in Advanced Cancer. *A Cancer Journal for Clinicians,* 51, 213–231

[8] Pott, M.; Haagen, M. et al. (2005). Wenn Mütter an Krebs erkranken: Seelische Auswirkungen auf Kinder und präventiver Handlungsbedarf. *Zentralblatt für Gynäkologie,* 127, 114–119

[9] Cartwright–Alcarese, F.; Sung, M.; Brenner, B.; Zambodla, A.; Geduld, A.; Desjardins, L. (2003). An Interdisciplinary Approach to the Provision of Patient Support Resources across the Oncology Care Continuum: Description of a Performance Improvement Project. *Journal of Nursing Care Quality,* 18 (1), 61–72

[10] Watson, M.; St. James-Roberts, I.; Ashley, S.; Tilney, C.; Brougham, B.; Edwards, L.; Baldus, C.; Romer, G. (2006). Factors associated with emotional and behavioural problems among school age children of breast cancer patients. *British Journal of Cancer,* 94, 43-50

[11] Morris, M. ; Grant, M.; Lynch, J. (2007). Patient-reported Family Distress Among Long-term Cancer Survivors. *Cancer Nursing,* 30(1), 1-8

[12] Hiddemann, W.; Huber, H.; Bartram, K. (2004). Die Onkologie- Teil 1- *Epidemiologie, Pathogenese, Grundprinzipien der Therapie,* Berlin-Heidelberg, Deutschland: Springer.

[13] Hasemann, W. (2006). Unterstützung (pflegender) Angehöriger in der Palliative Care. In Knipping, C. (Eds.), *Lehrbuch Palliative Care.* (1, 372-379). Bern: Hans Huber Verlag

[14] Teschendorf, B.; Schwartz, C.; Ferrans, C. E.; O´Mara, A.; Novotny, P.; Sloan, J. (2007). Caregiver role Stress: When Families Become Providers. *Cancer Control,* 14(2), 183-189

[15] Geigges, W. (2004). Krebs und Familie. *Psychoneuro,* 30 (4), 215-217

[16] Kaufmann, M. ; Ernst, B. (2000). CAWAC - Umfrage in Deutschland: Was Frauen mit Krebs erfahren, empfinden, wissen und vermissen. *Deutsches Ärzteblatt*, 97(4), 3191-3194

[17] Plant, H.: The impact of cancer on the family. (2001) In: Corner, J.; Bailey, C. (Eds.), *Cancer Nursing Care in Context.* (1, 86-99). London: Blackwell Science

[18] Lewis, F.; Woods, N.; Hough, E.; Bensley, L. (1989). The Family's Functioning With Chronic Illness In the Mother: The Spouse's Perspective. *Social Science Medcine,* 29 (11), 1261-1269

[19] Duhamel, F.; Dupuis, F. (2004). Guaranteed returns: investing in conversations with families of patients with cancer. *Clinical Journal of Oncology Nursing,* 8 (1), 68–71

[20] Friedemann, M. (1996). Familien- und umweltbezogene Pflege: die Theorie des systematischen Gleichgewichts, Bern, Schweiz: Hans Huber Verlag

[21] Krüger, C. (2006), Das WHO Konzept der Family Health Nurse in Deutschland: Möglichkeiten und Grenzen, Eine Literaturanalyse. Unveröffentlichtes Manuskript, Institut für Pflegewissenschaft, Universität Witten/Herdecke

[22] Wibmer, W.; Rechenberg-Winter, R. (2002). Paar- und Familientherapie. Manual Psychoonkologie, Tumorzentrum München, abgerufen im Internet unter: http://www.krebsinfo.de/ki/empfehlung/supportiv/732-40-Behrends.pdf (21.7.2007)

[23] Stetz, K. (2001) Lebensqualität in Familien mit tumorkranken Angehörigen. In King, C., Hinds, P. (Eds), Lebensqualität Pflege- und Patientenperspektive. Theorie – Forschung –Praxis (1,229-251) Bern: Hans Huber Verlag

[24] Leppin, C. (2006). Begleitung von Kindern und Jugendlichen als Angehörige schwer kranker Familienmitglieder In Knipping, C. (Eds.), *Lehrbuch Palliative Care,* (1,402-409) Bern: Hans Huber Verlag

[25] Koldjeski, D.; Kirkpatrick, M.; Everett, L.; Brown, S.; Swanson, M. (2007). The Ovarian Cancer Journey of Families- The first Postdiagnostic Year, *Cancer Nursing,* 30(3), 232-242

[26] Pro Familia Bundesverband (Eds.). Sexualität und Krebs (1999), abgerufen im Internet unter: http://www.profamilia.de/getpic/1656.pdf (Stand: 21.7.2007)

[27] Demnison, S. Sexuality and cancer (2001). In: Corner, J.; Bailey, C. (Eds.), Cancer Nursing Care in Context, (1, 420-428) London: Blackwell Science

[28] Weiland, S. (2007). Traumatisiert durch die Krankheit der Eltern, Ein innovatives Familien-Interventionsprogramm am Universitätskrankenhaus Eppendorf hilft Kindern, deren Mütter oder Väter schwer bis unheilbar erkrankt sind, abgerufen im www unter: http://www.aerztlichepraxis.de/artikel_paediatrie_psyche_cosip_1144682202.htm (Stand 23.7.2007)

[29] Forrest, G.; Plumb, C.; Zienbland, S.; Stein, A. (2006). Breast Cancer in the family-children's perceptions of their mother's cancer and its initial treatment: qualitative study. *British Medical Journal,* 332, 998-1003

[30] Barnes, J.; Kroll, L.; Burke, O.; Lee, J.; Jones, A.; Stein, A. (2000). Qualitative interview study of communication between parents and children about maternal breast cancer. *British Medical Journal,* 321, 479–482

[31] Zimmermann, A. (2002). Krankheitsverarbeitung und psychosoziales Umfeld. Manual Psychoonkologie. Tumorzentrum München. http://www.krebsinfo.de/ki/ empfehlung/ psychoo/787-05-Zimmermann.pdf (Stand: 10.7.2007)

[32] Huizinga, G., v. d. Graaf, W., Visser, A., Dijkstra, J., Hoekstra-Weebers, J.: Psychosocial Consequences for Children of a Parent with Cancer: A Pilot Study (2003). *Cancer Nursing,* 26(3), 195-202

[33] Haagen, M. (2004). Konflikte und Entwicklungsprobleme von Kindern schwer körperlich erkrankter Eltern, 39. Kongress der Ärztekammer Nordwürttemberg, Stuttgart 30.1.-1.2.2004 (Vortrag). www.aerztekmmer-bw.de/25/15medizin04/319/4.pdf.

[34] Kristjanson, L.; Chalmers, K.; Woodgate, R.: Information and Support Needs of Adolescent Children of Women with Breast Cancer (2004). *Oncology Nursing Forum,* 31(1), 111–118

[35] Schwarz, R.; Hornburg, E. (2001). Bewältigungsstrategien (Coping) bei Tumorerkrankungen. In Margulies, A.; Fellinger, K.; Gaisser, A.; Kroner, T. (Eds.), *Onkologische Krankenpflege.* (2001), (1, 219-229), Berlin: Springer

[36] Kylmä, J.; Vehviläinen-Julkunen, K. (2001). Eine Metaanalyse der ontologischen und epistemologischen Grundlagen der Hoffnung in der Pflegeforschung. In Schröck, R.; Drerup, E. (Eds.), Hoffen und Bangen, Beiträge der Pflegeforschung zu existentiellen Erfahrungen kranker Menschen und ihrer Angehörigen (2001), (1, 234-249) Freiburg im Breisgau: Lambertus Verlag

[37] Friesen, P.; Pepler, C.; Hunter, P. (2002). Interactive family learning following a cancer diagnosis. *Oncology Nursing Forum,* 29 (6), 981–987

[38] Eicher Ngochalit, M. (2004). Familienzentrierte Pflege –Ein Überblick Download: http://www.lindenhof-schule.ch/lh2/_data/1_publikationen_2jDGXGgmvXK6.pdf?ses=cf313972e2377866991dce01db6dd3d2 (Stand: 21.7.2007)

[39] Rolland, J. (2005). Cancer and the Family: An Integrative Model. *Cancer.* 104(S11), 2584-2595

[40] Knipping, C. (2006). Lehrbuch Bern: Hans Huber Verlag

[41] Blanchard, C.; Allbrecht, T.; Ruckdeschel, J. (1997). The Crisis of Cancer: Psychological Impact on Family Caregivers. *Oncology,* 11 (2), 189–194

[42] Abt-Zegelin, A. (2000) In Walsh, M.; Ford, P.; Abt - Zegelin, A. (Eds.). *Pflegerituale,* Bern: Hans Huber Verlag

Index

A

AC, 91
academic performance, 48
academic success, 47
access, 16, 17, 45
accidents, 133
accommodation, 63, 64, 72
accounting, 37
accuracy, vii, 7, 10, 16
achievement, 33, 37, 45, 46
achievement orientation, 37
action research, 105
activation, 66
acute stress, 32, 63, 65, 66
adaptability, 38
adaptation, vii, 23, 24, 25, 26, 37, 43, 44, 45, 47, 50, 51, 54, 55, 59, 72, 74, 109, 126
adaptive functioning, 43, 44
ADHD, 46, 47, 54, 55
adjustment, viii, 11, 23, 24, 25, 26, 27, 28, 29, 30, 31, 32, 33, 34, 35, 36, 38, 39, 41, 42, 43, 44, 45, 46, 47, 49, 50, 54, 56, 57, 58, 59, 60, 69, 71, 75, 79, 87, 91, 92, 93, 109, 126
adolescents, 27, 36, 38, 39, 52, 53, 57, 58, 59, 135
adulthood, 31, 33, 50
adults, 33, 41, 56, 125
adverse event, 18, 20
advocacy, 4, 50
aetiology, 133, 135
affective reactions, 34, 53
African American women, 19
afternoon, 98
age, vii, 1, 26, 29, 30, 33, 34, 35, 45, 53, 58, 82, 87, 112, 124, 128, 133, 134, 138
agent, 3, 56
aggressiveness, 39
alcohol, 37
algorithm, 14
alopecia, 129
alternative(s), 14, 18, 19, 71, 79, 96, 109, 111, 123, 125, 126, 134
alternative medicine, 14, 109, 111, 125, 126
alters, vii, 61, 62
ambiguity, 33, 104
ambivalence, 47, 90
American Cancer Society, 24, 51
American Psychiatric Association, 40, 51, 63, 73
American Psychological Association, 59, 76
anger, vii, 35, 39, 68, 71, 80, 81, 82, 83, 85, 88, 92, 110, 123
ANOVA, 89, 114
anthroposophic, x, xi,107, 108, 111, 113, 114, 115, 116, 117, 118, 120, 121, 122, 123, 124, 125
antibody, 16
anxiety, vii, ix, 2, 24, 26, 27, 28, 32, 33, 35, 36, 39, 40, 41, 56, 63, 66, 72, 77, 78, 79, 80, 81, 82, 83, 84, 85, 86, 87, 88, 90, 91, 92, 128, 131, 134, 135
anxiety reaction, 82
anxiousness, 110
AP, 113
appetite, 113
appraisals, 35
AR, 105
arousal, ix, 61, 63, 68, 72
articulation, 104
ASD, 66
assessment, 9, 14, 15, 27, 40, 42, 50, 78, 91, 93, 110, 136

assessment tools, 50
assimilation, 63, 64, 72
assumptions, 71, 74, 124
astrocytoma, 56
asymmetry, 104
attachment, 43, 67
attention, 29, 42, 46, 47, 51, 63, 67, 68, 73, 103, 104, 128
attitudes, x, 48, 77, 79, 87, 92
attribution, 53
Australia, 2, 4, 5, 11, 57
autonomy, x, 33, 65, 95, 96, 99, 100, 103, 104
availability, 17, 46, 68
avoidance, 26, 32, 35, 37, 40, 45, 63, 68, 72, 79, 85
awareness, 34, 48, 67, 69, 71, 103, 130, 137

B

batteries, 98
behavior, x, 8, 26, 28, 31, 34, 36, 37, 38, 39, 40, 45, 50, 52, 58, 77, 80, 81, 87, 88, 90, 100
behavior therapy, 87, 88, 90
behavioral change, 51
beliefs, 33, 34, 55, 57
benefits, 37, 110
benign, 47, 78, 80, 91
bias, 11
biological processes, 20
biomarkers, 20
biopsy, 82, 83
birth, 37, 45, 59, 60
birth weight, 37
bladder, 29
blame, 44, 132
blood, 29, 75, 137
body fluid, 20
body image, 3
bone marrow transplant, 65
bone tumors, 56
borrowing, 47
brain, 29, 30, 31, 39, 47, 52, 60, 67, 73, 74, 75
brain development, 29, 30
brain tumor, 30, 31, 39, 52, 60, 73, 74
BRCA1, 14, 16
BRCA2, 16
breast, vii, 1, 2, 3, 4, 5, 91, 107, 108, 126, 138, 139, 140
breast cancer, vii, x, 1, 2, 3, 4, 5, 9, 11, 16, 19, 79, 80, 81, 87, 90, 91, 92, 107, 108, 109, 110, 111, 123, 124, 125, 126, 138, 139
breast mass, 91
breathing, 101, 102
burnout, 69, 74
business model, viii, 13, 18

C

cancer care, 4, 96, 104
cancer cells, 67
cancer progression, 108
cancer treatment, ix, 29, 56, 61, 62, 64, 65, 66, 68, 69, 74, 75, 108, 110
carcinoma, 11
cardiomyopathy, 29
care model, 73
caregivers, x, 36, 40, 41, 45, 50, 51, 52, 55, 57, 62, 95, 96, 97, 104, 105, 128, 129
caregiving, 33, 40, 41, 44, 48, 74
carrier, 18
catalyst, 35
causal attribution, 34
cell, 11, 20, 26, 27, 35, 37, 58, 59, 75
cell transplantation, 75
central nervous system, 29, 30, 73, 131
certainty, 35, 108
Chalmers, 140
chemotherapy, viii, 13, 18, 29, 30, 52, 53, 99, 101, 103, 110, 112
Chicago, 57
child development, 34, 35, 50
child well-being, 28, 31
childhood, ix, 11, 24, 25, 26, 27, 28, 29, 31, 32, 33, 35, 36, 37, 38, 39, 40, 41, 42, 46, 47, 52, 53, 54, 55, 56, 57, 58, 59, 60, 61, 62, 63, 64, 65, 66, 67, 68, 69, 70, 72, 73, 74, 75, 76
childhood disorders, 57
child-rearing practices, 74
children, ix, xi,23, 24, 25, 26, 27, 28, 29, 30, 31, 32, 33, 34, 35, 36, 37, 38, 39, 40, 41, 42, 43, 44, 45, 46, 47, 48, 49, 50, 51, 52, 53, 54, 55, 56, 57, 58, 59, 60, 61, 62, 64, 65, 66, 67, 68, 70, 73, 74, 75, 112, 127, 128, 130, 132, 133, 134, 135, 136, 137, 138, 139
chronic illness, ix, 23, 24, 25, 26, 27, 28, 32, 35, 36, 37, 39, 41, 42, 43, 44, 50, 51, 57, 137
chronic myelogenous, 19
chronic stress, ix, 24, 25, 40, 50, 61, 66, 68
cleaning, 101
clinical assessment, 50
clinical psychology, 47

close relationships, 31
clusters, 63, 68
CNS, 3, 29
coaches, 70
coding, 9, 10
cognition, 53
cognitive development, 35, 55, 132
cognitive dissonance, 70
cognitive flexibility, 47
cognitive function, 35, 113, 115
cognitive performance, 46
cognitive process, 26, 59, 110
cognitive therapy, 80
cohesion, 37, 38, 45
cohesiveness, 49
cohort, 126
collaboration, 62, 73
communication, xi,4, 37, 48, 74, 92, 98, 104, 127, 130, 131, 133, 134, 136, 137, 139
community, 11, 17, 19, 31, 38, 50, 51, 66
community support, 19
compassion, 72
competence, 44, 57
competency, 92
complexity, 33, 51, 128
compliance, 19
complications, 17, 56, 73, 102
components, 47
computers, 9
computing, 9
conceptualization, 46
concrete, 68, 103
confidence, 48, 50, 64, 88
conflict, 27, 33, 37, 70, 103
confrontation, 37
confusion, 47, 82, 83, 85
Connecticut, 77
consciousness, 70
consensus, 108
consent, 82, 87
constipation, 113
construct validity, 39
construction, 11, 30, 62
content analysis, 10
control, 20, 26, 27, 34, 35, 36, 37, 38, 44, 48, 50, 64, 65, 70, 80, 89, 92, 100, 104, 129
control group, 36, 48, 89
controlled trials, 19
convergence, 19, 20, 36
coping model, ix, 23, 24, 25, 26, 27, 42, 50
coping strategies, xi,8, 27, 36, 37, 44, 45, 54, 109, 110, 125, 126, 127, 135, 136
coping strategy, 35, 39, 109, 113, 123
correlation(s), 39, 82, 83, 84, 85, 86
correlation coefficient, 83, 84, 85, 86
costs, 17, 18, 128
counseling, 1, 3, 4, 5, 48
counterbalance, 65
couples, 36, 53, 65, 130
credibility, 97
criticism, 64
CRP, 47
crying, 36
CT scan, 17, 20
culture, 104
cycling, 99
cystic fibrosis, 26, 27, 59
cytokines, 75

D

daily care, 100
daily living, 45
data collection, 112, 116, 118, 120, 122, 123
death, vii, ix, 16, 61, 62, 63, 70, 71, 74, 75, 77, 79, 90, 110, 132, 133, 136
decision makers, 48
decision making, 75, 137
decisions, vii, 64, 68, 70, 98, 104, 137
defects, 63, 67
defensiveness, 108
deficit(s), 24, 29, 30, 31, 32, 42, 46, 47, 49, 51, 53, 67
definition, 3, 8, 39, 64
delivery, 14
demand, 18, 38, 66
demographic factors, 27, 37
demographics, 15, 31
denial, 63, 78, 93, 110, 131
Department of Health and Human Services, 16
depression, vii, ix, 27, 28, 32, 33, 35, 36, 40, 44, 72, 77, 78, 79, 80, 81, 82, 83, 85, 90, 92, 110, 123
depressive symptoms, 40, 90, 91
desires, 97
detachment, 71
detection, viii, 2, 5, 14, 17, 19
developing countries, 62
developmental process, 33, 34
diabetes, 41
diagnostic criteria, 40

diarrhea, 99, 113
diet, 14, 40, 113
disability, 24, 31, 42, 43, 44, 45, 46, 47, 49, 50, 51, 52, 54, 55, 57
disappointment, 32
discipline, 9
disclosure, ix, x, 36, 49, 57, 61, 62, 63, 64, 66, 77, 82, 83, 84, 85, 86, 87, 88, 90
discomfort, 131
disease progression, 20, 29
disorder, 33, 40, 46, 51, 54, 63, 66, 68
dissatisfaction, 42, 89
distress, viii, x, 2, 8, 23, 24, 26, 27, 28, 30, 31, 32, 34, 35, 36, 39, 40, 43, 44, 48, 49, 56, 58, 62, 65, 66, 72, 73, 74, 75, 76, 77, 78, 79, 80, 81, 82, 86, 89, 90, 91, 92, 107, 109, 111, 126
distribution, 114
divergence, 20
diversity, 15, 19, 37
doctors, 98, 101, 104
dominance, 98
dosage, 18
dosing, 70
drugs, 18, 19, 70
DSM, 40, 73
DSM-IV, 73
duration, ix, 61, 62, 135
duties, 128
dyspnea, 70, 113

E

eating, 15, 40
eating disorder, 133
economic status, 15, 31, 32, 45
education, vii, 1, 3, 19, 30, 42, 47, 49, 50, 56, 57, 60, 89, 90, 105, 108
educational psychology, 47
educational services, 47, 50
educational system, 48, 50
emerging issues, 97
emotion(s), vii, ix, x, 7, 8, 9, 10, 11, 32, 36, 37, 38, 44, 45, 49, 53, 55, 68, 70, 71, 72, 77, 80, 81, 83, 86, 87, 88, 89, 90, 92, 97, 107, 109, 124, 135
emotional disorder, 80, 91
emotional distress, 48, 80, 81, 92
emotional experience, 32, 40
emotional reactions, 75
emotional well-being, 29
employees, 112
employment, ix, 56, 61, 65
empowerment, 104
encouragement, 31
endocrine, 28, 29, 30, 66, 67, 74
energy, 32, 42, 66, 100, 134
England, 52
enlargement, 48
environment, 18, 20, 26, 30, 34, 35
environmental factors, 25
equilibrium, 32
equipment, 129
ethical questions, x, 95
ethics, 105
evening, 98
evidence, 5, 24, 26, 28, 34, 35, 36, 38, 39, 40, 41, 43, 46, 47, 48, 49, 50, 52, 57, 108, 123
evolution, 15
exclusion, 89
exercise, 14, 40, 47
expenditures, 17
expertise, 102
exposure, 15, 66, 69
external locus of control, 44
externalizing behavior, 26

F

facial expression, 9
factor analysis, 39, 55
failure, 30, 62
faith, 69
family, vii, ix, x, xi,1, 14, 15, 20, 23, 24, 25, 26, 27, 28, 31, 32, 33, 34, 35, 36, 37, 38, 39, 40, 43, 44, 45, 48, 50, 51, 52, 53, 54, 55, 56, 57, 58, 59, 60, 61, 62, 63, 65, 67, 68, 70, 72, 74, 77, 78, 90, 95, 96, 97, 98, 100, 103, 104, 105, 110, 113, 115, 127, 128, 129, 130, 132, 133, 134, 135, 136, 137, 139, 140
family conflict, 27, 37, 133
family factors, 57
family functioning, ix, 23, 24, 26, 27, 33, 34, 37, 38, 39, 43, 44, 45, 50, 53, 54, 55, 57, 58, 59
family history, 14, 15
family life, xi,51, 127, 130
family members, vii, 1, 38, 45, 62, 100, 103, 104, 128, 130, 136, 137
family relationships, 31, 35
family structures, 128
family support, 27, 28, 37, 44, 54
family system, 24, 25, 54

family therapy, 48
fatalism, 79, 80, 85, 86, 90, 110
fatalistic, x, 77, 79, 80
fatigue, 30, 69, 70, 74, 82, 83, 85, 113, 129
FDA, 15, 18
fear, vii, ix, 32, 63, 65, 68, 77, 78, 88, 90, 97, 134
fears, viii, 23, 24, 32, 49, 79, 131, 133
federal law, 30
feedback, 19, 87
feelings, vii, 32, 33, 35, 36, 37, 43, 48, 51, 64, 66, 68, 69, 71, 72, 81, 87, 97, 104, 128, 129, 133, 134
fever, 132
fibrosis, 26, 27, 59
financial stability, 45
financial support, 33
Finland, 124
flexibility, 24, 38, 47, 49
flight, 66
fluid, 20, 99
focusing, 37, 64, 110
Ford, 140
foreclosure, 33
forgiveness, 72
formal education, vii, 1, 3
fragility, 32, 105
friendship, 31
frustration, 42
fulfillment, 44
futures, 33

G

gender, 26, 29, 30
gene, 16
gene expression, 16
general practitioner, 15, 96, 97, 103
genome, 16
genotype, 16
genre, x, 95
Germany, xi,127, 128, 132, 137
gland, 101
goals, 5, 7, 31, 33, 48, 97
God, 36
grants, 124
grief, ix, 3, 29, 32, 42, 48, 50, 61, 63, 69, 71, 72, 73, 75
groups, x, 9, 11, 17, 19, 27, 28, 36, 45, 47, 48, 53, 89, 95, 97, 113, 115, 116, 118, 120, 123, 130, 131
growth, viii, 7, 30, 34, 35, 43, 44, 50, 64, 67, 69, 72, 73, 75
guidance, 19, 49, 69
guidelines, 2, 10, 16
guilt, vii, 35, 39, 68, 69, 71
guilty, 129, 133

H

hair loss, 64
hands, 78, 90
happiness, 44
health, viii, 3, 5, 10, 14, 17, 23, 24, 26, 27, 29, 31, 33, 36, 38, 39, 40, 41, 45, 48, 49, 53, 55, 56, 58, 59, 64, 67, 73, 74, 75, 91, 92, 96, 97, 103, 105, 108, 123, 124, 126, 128, 129, 130, 136, 137
Health and Human Services, 16
health care, 3, 17, 38, 53, 56, 64, 74, 97, 103, 128, 129, 136, 137
health care costs, 17
health care professionals, 3, 103, 137
health care system, 128, 129
health locus of control, 26
health problems, 31
health status, 31, 53, 126
hearing loss, 29
heart attack, 98
helplessness, x, 33, 35, 66, 77, 78, 79, 80, 81, 86, 110
herceptin, 16
high fat, 80
higher quality, xi,108, 115, 120, 122, 123, 124
hip, 44
holistic care, 113
hopelessness, x, 71, 77, 78, 79, 80, 81, 86, 110
hospice, 105
hospitalization, 17, 87
hospitals, 40
host, 20
hostility, 82, 85
households, 45
human development, 52
humanity, 81
husband, 103
hyperactivity, 51
hypothesis, 36
hysterectomy, 131

I

identification, 10, 17, 18, 96

identity, 33, 71, 128
identity achievement, 33
images, 72
imaging, 17, 18, 20
immune function, 40, 55
immunity, 54, 55
impairments, ix, 30, 31, 46, 47, 61
implementation, ix, 14, 24, 25, 98
impulsivity, 46
in situ, 129
inclusion, xi,104, 108, 112
income, 31
independence, 37
indication, viii, 13, 15
indicators, 11
industry, 18, 19
inertia, 82
infancy, 53
infants, 37
infectious disease, 40, 52
infertility, 29, 67, 131
inflammatory, 75
information processing, 63, 64
information seeking, 36, 110, 123
informed consent, 82, 87
inhibition, 92
injections, 99
injury(ies), 29, 47, 131
injustice, 68
insight, 32, 48, 68
institutions, 3, 18
instruction, 47
instruments, 83, 87, 124
insurance, 17, 56
integrity, 45
intellectual disabilities, 44, 47, 48, 54
intellectual functioning, 58
intensity, vii, ix, 7, 31, 33, 61, 66
intentions, 8
interaction(s), 14, 19, 25, 31, 34, 39, 43, 45, 65
internalizing, 26, 28, 33
internet, 14, 18, 19, 77, 139
interpersonal relationships, 48
interpretation, 96, 97, 105, 133
intervention, viii, x, 8, 11, 13, 14, 15, 16, 17, 18, 20, 23, 25, 26, 29, 30, 36, 37, 47, 48, 49, 50, 53, 54, 75, 77, 80, 86, 87, 88, 89, 90
interview, 78, 97, 139
intrusions, 63, 68
inventions, 49
investment, 17
iPod, viii, 14
irradiation, 30
irritability, 39
isolation, 68, 132, 133
Israel, 1, 3, 5

J

Japan, 77, 90, 92
judgment, 31

K

kidney, 29
King, 139

L

lack of control, 129
language, 9, 97, 99
laws, 30
lead, ix, 8, 15, 21, 47, 61, 64, 67, 72, 128, 130, 134, 135
learning, ix, x, 23, 24, 25, 30, 31, 41, 42, 43, 45, 46, 47, 48, 49, 50, 51, 52, 53, 55, 59, 62, 63, 65, 77, 90, 96, 102, 140
learning behavior, 52
learning disabilities, ix, 23, 24, 25, 30, 42, 45, 46, 47, 48, 50, 51, 53, 55
learning process, 96
leukemia, 19, 29, 52, 54, 55, 73, 74
life cycle, 51, 131
life expectancy, 78
life satisfaction, 124, 125
lifestyle, 14, 15, 32
limitation, 124
linear model, 63
linguistics, vii, 7, 9, 10
linkage, 16, 34
links, 92, 103
listening, 101
literature, 3, 24, 33, 42, 43, 50, 52, 58, 105, 109, 129
living conditions, 131
localization, 18, 112
location, 29, 30
locus, 26, 44, 49, 50
London, 4, 5, 125, 139
loneliness, 32, 70, 72

longitudinal study(ies), x, 26, 27, 37, 38, 40, 53, 107, 111, 124
low risk, 14, 15
lung, 79, 91
lung cancer, 79, 91
lying, 132

M

males, 31
malignant tumors, 29, 30
management, viii, 4, 13, 14, 15, 16, 19, 21, 33, 48, 65, 70, 91, 103, 104, 130, 136
marital discord, 65
marital status, 56
market, 18
marriage, 31, 42, 102
married couples, 130
marrow, 65, 74
MAS, 82, 83, 84, 85
Massachusetts, 11
mastectomy, 5, 14, 16, 131
meanings, 10, 97, 100
measurement, 10, 21, 28, 56
measures, vii, 2, 7, 8, 39, 46, 47, 49, 66, 79, 80, 87, 108
median, 87, 114
medical care, 29, 64, 73, 75, 137
medication, 14, 19, 46, 52, 136
medicine, 14, 15, 16, 18, 19, 109, 111, 114, 123, 125, 126
memory, 29, 30, 53, 67
meningitis, 29, 63
mental disorder, 73
mental health, 27, 33, 40, 41, 48, 49
messages, 88, 133
meta-analysis, 9, 49, 56, 110, 126
metaphor, 99
metastasis, 112
methylphenidate, 46, 47, 54, 55, 56, 59
Ministry of Education, 90
minority, 26, 67, 68
MIT, 11
models, 8, 25, 42, 46, 63, 72
money, 132
mood, 2, 36, 82, 85
morbidity, 2, 5, 17, 80, 91, 93
morning, 102
mortality, 40, 57
mortality risk, 40
mothers, 27, 28, 29, 31, 32, 36, 37, 39, 40, 43, 44, 49, 50, 52, 53, 54, 55, 56, 57, 58, 59, 73, 76, 132, 133
motor function, 67
MRI, 17
multidimensional, ix, x, 23, 45, 107, 110
muscular dystrophy, 59
mutation, 14
mutations, 16

N

narratives, 10, 11
nasogastric tube, 101, 102
nausea, 113, 129
negative affectivity, 36
negative emotions, x, 11, 77, 81, 88, 89
negative outcomes, 34, 36
nervous system, 29, 30, 73, 131
Netherlands, 57, 95, 96, 101
network, 45
networking, 14, 19
New England, 52
New York, 11, 51, 52, 55, 56, 74, 75, 91, 92, 125
New Zealand, 57
North America, 3, 5, 76
Norway, 111, 126
nurses, x, xi,2, 3, 4, 5, 95, 96, 98, 99, 100, 101, 102, 103, 104, 127, 136, 138
nursing, vii, xi,1, 3, 4, 96, 97, 100, 103, 105, 127, 128, 129, 130, 136, 137
nursing care, 128, 129, 130, 136
nursing home, 97, 103

O

obesity, 65, 67
observations, 133
oncology, 2, 4, 5, 11, 53, 55, 56, 57, 59, 60, 73, 74, 75, 91, 92, 125, 126, 138, 139, 140
openness, 37
optimism, 71, 90, 135
organization(s), 2, 3, 37, 97, 103
orientation, 34, 37
osteoporosis, 29
outcome relationship, 25
outpatients, 80
overload, 73

P

Pacific, 74
pain, viii, ix, 13, 26, 27, 40, 61, 64, 70, 72, 74, 101, 113, 131
pain management, 70
pain therapy, 101
palliative, viii, x, 13, 20, 21, 26, 27, 28, 35, 36, 95, 96, 97, 100, 103, 104, 105, 128
palliative care, viii, x, 13, 95, 96, 100, 103, 105, 128
pap smear, 10
parenting, 24, 25, 28, 29, 30, 31, 32, 33, 35, 38, 39, 40, 41, 42, 43, 44, 45, 46, 47, 48, 49, 50, 53, 58, 65
parents, viii, ix, 23, 24, 25, 28, 29, 30, 31, 32, 33, 34, 35, 36, 37, 38, 39, 40, 41, 42, 43, 44, 45, 46, 47, 48, 49, 50, 51, 53, 54, 55, 57, 58, 59, 60, 61, 62, 63, 64, 65, 66, 67, 68, 69, 70, 71, 72, 73, 74, 75, 128, 130, 132, 133, 134, 139
particles, 18
partnership(s), xi,127, 131, 137
passive, 64, 81, 100, 113
patient care, 14, 19, 21
patient management, 4
pediatric, viii, 23, 24, 25, 29, 36, 38, 39, 41, 42, 46, 47, 49, 50, 51, 52, 56, 57, 60, 73, 74, 75, 76
peer relationship, 60
peers, 31, 33
percentile, 43
perception(s), 31, 35, 44, 45, 54, 56, 66, 72, 74, 110, 126, 128, 136, 139
performance, viii, 13, 29, 46, 47, 48, 67
personal, viii, 14, 19, 21, 34, 35, 37, 43, 44, 48, 50, 69, 70, 71, 72, 75, 80, 96, 97, 99, 103, 104
personal achievements, 70
personal responsibility, 35
personality, 78, 86, 91, 101
personality traits, 78
PET, 17, 20
pharmacology, 52
physical health, 24, 31, 40, 41
pilot study, 10, 57
placebo, 47, 56
planning, 14, 36, 105
plasma, 19
plasma levels, 19
PM, 105
poison, 99
polarity, 69
poor, 27, 28, 29, 31, 34, 38, 40, 41, 72, 80, 110
population, viii, xi,8, 9, 14, 15, 23, 24, 27, 28, 29, 31, 40, 41, 42, 46, 47, 48, 49, 50, 125, 126, 127
positive correlation, 39
positive relationship, 39
post traumatic stress disorder, 40
posttraumatic stress, 34, 48, 54, 57, 73, 76
post-traumatic stress disorder (PTSD), 33, 40, 54, 63, 66, 68, 72
power, 103
predictability, ix, 61, 62
prediction, 15
predictors, viii, 11, 16, 23, 32, 44, 50, 125
premature death, 16
preparedness, 47, 135
pressure, 71, 103
prevention, 16, 17, 25, 91, 130
primary caregivers, 51, 52, 105
probability, 15, 16, 63, 79, 133, 134
problem solving, 35, 36, 44
problem-focused coping, 8, 26, 44, 109, 110, 126
problem-solver, 70
problem-solving, 36, 48, 50
problem-solving behavior, 36
problem-solving skills, 36
production, 52
profession, vii, xi,1, 3, 127, 130, 137
prognosis, 33, 63, 79, 80, 92, 112, 124, 125, 130, 135
program, viii, 9, 10, 13, 14, 48, 113
programming, 10
pro-inflammatory, 75
promote, 9, 48, 51, 64
prophylactic, 16
prostate cancer, 125
protocol, 8
psychiatric morbidity, 2, 5, 79, 91
psychological distress, x, 33, 44, 49, 56, 77, 78, 79, 80, 81, 82, 86, 89, 90, 91, 92, 107, 109
psychological illnesses, 132
psychological problems, 109, 123
psychological processes, ix, 61, 62
psychological resources, 130
psychological stress, 75
psychological variables, 90
psychological well-being, 31
psychology, 9, 10, 47, 74
psychometric properties, 124
psychopathology, 25, 32

psychosocial, viii, 1, 2, 9, 23, 25, 26, 27, 31, 32, 33, 36, 37, 50, 51, 54, 55, 57, 60, 74, 78, 80, 108, 111, 123, 125
psychosocial development, 33
psychosocial factors, 108
psychosocial functioning, 51, 54
psychosocial support, 33
psychosomatic, 52, 54, 55, 56,66, 91, 92, 138
psychotherapy, 92
punishment, 88

Q

QLQ-C30, x, 108, 113
qualifications, 102
quality improvement, x, 95
quality of life, viii, x, xi,4, 11, 13, 16, 21, 24, 30, 31, 33, 36, 40, 52, 53, 54, 67, 74, 75, 77, 80, 98, 100, 103, 104, 105, 107, 108, 109, 110, 111, 113, 114, 115, 116, 117, 118, 119, 120, 121, 122, 123, 124, 125, 126, 131
questioning, 33, 68, 70
questionnaire(s), 74, 79, 82, 83, 92, 93, 103, 124, 125, 126

R

radiation, 15, 18, 29, 30, 50, 74, 110
radiation therapy, 29, 30, 74
radical mastectomy, 14
radiotherapy, viii, 13, 112
rain, 31
range, vii, 7, 8, 20, 27, 37, 62, 65, 71, 72, 82, 87, 100, 113
ratings, 46, 60, 91
reaction time, 46
reading, 9, 20, 97, 105, 132
reality, viii, 14, 16, 32, 35, 62, 63, 133, 135
recognition, 18, 25, 63
recovery, 21, 67, 69, 73, 110
recurrence, viii, x, 15, 23, 24, 32, 67, 69, 77, 78, 79, 90
reduction, 25, 46, 47, 48, 131, 134
reflection, 33, 98, 100
reforms, 18
regional, 96, 97, 113
regulation(s), 30, 75
regulatory requirements, 19
rehabilitation, 47, 69
reinforcement, 43
relationship(s), x, 3, 19, 25, 29, 30, 31, 33, 34, 35, 37, 38, 39, 41, 43, 44, 45, 48, 54, 58, 60, 65, 72, 78, 79, 81, 82, 83, 85, 92, 95, 101, 102, 104, 113, 128, 130, 131, 134, 135
relatives, 71, 96, 105
relaxation, 48
relevance, 103
reliability, 9, 39, 91, 93, 124
religion, 36, 110
remediation, 52
renal cell carcinoma, 11
resection, 18, 30
resentment, 35
resilience, 42
resistance, 75
resolution, 17, 20
resources, 3, 24, 31, 38, 39, 43, 44, 45, 47, 48, 49, 57, 63, 64, 65, 109, 130, 135, 136, 137
respiratory, 52
restructuring, 34, 48, 69, 110, 123
returns, 139
Reynolds, 52
RF, 113, 115
risk, viii, 14, 15, 16, 23, 24, 25, 29, 30, 31, 35, 37, 40, 41, 43, 56, 57, 65, 67, 71, 80, 82, 86, 124, 129, 132, 133
risk assessment, 15
risk factors, 82, 86, 133
romantic relationship, 31
routines, 100, 132

S

sadness, vii, ix, 32, 77, 88, 90
safety, 16, 18, 20
salt, 99
sample, 11, 32, 33, 37, 38, 41, 44, 45, 46, 115, 124, 126
satisfaction, 44, 45, 48, 124, 125, 131
Scandinavia, 2
scheduling, 8
school, 30, 31, 32, 42, 43, 45, 51, 53, 55, 67, 132, 133, 138
school performance, 67
science, 128, 137
scores, xi,36, 43, 82, 83, 85, 87, 89, 108, 113, 126
search, 19
searching, 71
secondary education, 42

seizures, 30
self esteem, 30, 44
self-assessment, 40
self-concept, 53
self-confidence, 48
self-control, 44
self-efficacy, 26, 50
self-esteem, 26, 44, 48, 131
self-reports, 36
self-worth, 26
sensations, 131
sensitivity, 17, 20
separation, 72
series, viii, 2, 13, 97
SES, 113, 115
severe stress, ix, 61, 64, 66, 72
severity, 24, 26, 28, 33, 43, 50, 52, 102
sexual activities, 131
sexual violence, 131
sexuality, 3, 131
shame, 68, 69, 97
sharing, 45
shock, vii, 62, 63
sibling, 38, 53
siblings, ix, 31, 54, 59, 61, 65, 68, 70, 74
sickle cell, 26, 27, 37, 58, 59
side effects, 18, 33, 47, 62, 64, 134
signals, 19
signs, 15, 73, 132
similarity, 46, 47
sites, 14, 18, 19
skills, 31, 34, 36, 44, 46, 48, 57, 80, 81, 87, 101, 102, 135
skills training, 36, 57
skin, 99
sleep disturbance, ix, 61, 72, 113
smoking, 37
social activities, 45
social adjustment, 34
social competence, 57
social impairment, 31
social isolation, 132
social life, 67, 73
social network, 14, 19, 45
social perception, 31
social relationships, 30, 55
social roles, 31
social sciences, 10
social skills, 34, 46
social support, vii, 1, 33, 38, 43, 44, 45, 46, 47, 49, 50, 55, 56, 76, 78, 80, 92, 110, 123
socialization, 34, 53
society, 62
socioeconomic status, 26, 108, 109
special education, 47
specificity, 20
spectrum, 97, 128
speech, 9, 10
speed, 16, 47
spina bifida, 55
spirituality, 110
spousal relations, 44
SPSS, 114
stability, x, 26, 27, 45, 63, 64, 107, 111
stages, viii, 3, 14, 15, 49, 63
stakeholders, x, 20, 95, 96, 97, 104
statistics, 14, 114, 132
stethoscope, 101
stigma, 14
stimulant, 46, 52
stoma, 99
strain, ix, 40, 41, 61, 64, 65, 66, 71, 128, 129
strategies, xi,8, 18, 26, 27, 36, 37, 44, 45, 47, 48, 54, 75, 91, 109, 110, 125, 126, 127, 135, 136
strength, 44, 50, 60, 72, 124
stress, viii, ix, x, xi,23, 24, 25, 26, 27, 28, 30, 33, 34, 35, 36, 37, 38, 39, 40, 41, 42, 43, 44, 45, 46, 47, 48, 49, 50, 51, 52, 53, 54, 55, 56, 57, 58, 59, 61, 63, 64, 65, 66, 68, 69, 71, 73, 75, 76, 77, 81, 86, 88, 89, 90, 91, 107, 108, 109, 111, 127, 134
stress reactions, 66
stressful events, 33, 109
stressors, ix, 25, 28, 32, 38, 41, 42, 49, 50, 61, 62, 64, 65, 66, 67, 68, 69, 71, 72, 73, 75
suffering, 34, 64, 74, 100, 103, 135
summer, 36
suppression, x, 77, 80, 81, 82, 83, 86, 89, 90, 91, 92
surgical resection, 30
surplus, 74
surveillance, 14
survival, x, xi,19, 25, 48, 63, 107, 108, 110, 111, 120, 122, 123, 124, 125, 126
survival rate, 25, 63, 111
survivors, viii, 11, 23, 24, 25, 28, 29, 30, 31, 32, 33, 34, 35, 37, 38, 39, 40, 41, 42, 43, 46, 47, 48, 49, 50, 51, 52, 53, 54, 55, 56, 57, 59, 60, 64, 67, 68, 73, 75, 78, 91, 125
susceptibility, 52
Sweden, 61, 107, 124

symptomology, 39, 40
symptom(s), viii, ix, 13, 15, 26, 27, 31, 33, 34, 35, 36, 39, 40, 44, 48, 52, 53, 54, 61, 63, 66, 68, 69, 70, 72, 73, 90, 91, 104, 110, 113, 115, 129, 130, 131, 132, 133, 136
syndrome, 31, 66, 68, 69, 74
synthesis, 58
systems, 10, 25, 45, 54, 135

T

targets, viii, 18, 23, 25, 26, 27, 29
task performance, 47
teachers, 47
teaching, 33
technology, viii, 13, 16, 19, 20, 21, 40, 59, 70
teenagers, 65
telephone, 132
temporal lobe, 56
tension, 78, 82, 83
theoretical assumptions, 124
theory, 7, 11, 51, 63, 64, 104, 125
therapeutic, viii, 13, 18, 20, 34, 48, 49, 52, 68, 113, 127, 131, 137
therapeutic interventions, 18, 131
therapeutic targets, 18
therapeutics, 18
therapy, 11, 18, 19, 20, 29, 30, 33, 36, 48, 73, 74, 80, 87, 88, 90, 91, 92, 101, 113, 126, 128
thinking, 26, 35, 44, 72, 80, 88, 89, 90, 110
threat(s), 7, 63, 66, 67, 69, 70, 80
thyroid, 101
thyroid gland, 101
time elements, 20
tissue, 18
toxicity, 29
tracheostomy, 101
training, 36, 57, 67, 69
trait anxiety, 82, 86
traits, 78
trajectory, ix, 37, 38, 61, 68, 105
transactional stress, ix, 23, 24, 25, 42
transactions, 25
transformation(s), 68, 130
transition, 31, 33, 51, 73, 74
transition to adulthood, 31
transplantation, 74, 75
trauma, 32, 36, 63, 64, 74
traumatic events, 64, 66
traumatic experiences, ix, 61
trial, viii, x, 11, 13, 46, 56, 57, 78, 91
triggers, 34, 52, 69
trust, 102
tumor(s)s, 15, 17, 18, 19, 29, 30, 31, 39, 52, 53, 56, 60, 67, 73, 74, 75

U

UK, 1, 2, 3
ultrasound, 17
uncertainty, 29, 32, 33, 35, 39, 49, 52, 56, 57, 62, 63, 65, 66, 69, 72, 134
United Kingdom, 4
users, 109, 111

V

vaccine, 11
validation, 11, 17, 51, 52
validity, 10, 39, 92, 93, 124
values, 33, 97, 117, 119
variability, 24, 25, 28, 30, 31, 32, 34, 42, 43, 50, 72
variable(s), ix, 23, 24, 27, 34, 38, 42, 43, 47, 50, 54, 90, 91, 113, 123, 125
variance, 26, 27, 28, 37, 89, 114
variation, 27, 72
vehicles, 18
vein, 99
victims, 55
Victoria, 73
violence, 131
vision, 30
voice, 2, 97, 98
vomiting, 113
vulnerability, 78

W

walking, 99, 100
war, 99
Washington, 59, 73, 76
weakness, 81, 88
wealth, vii, 7
wear, 99
weight loss, 131
welfare, 100, 101
well-being, 1, 28, 29, 31, 41, 62, 67, 70, 75
wellness, 40, 41
western countries, 2, 3, 130

wetting, 133
wives, 44
women, vii, x, xi,1, 2, 3, 4, 5, 9, 11, 19, 40, 80, 90, 91, 92, 107, 108, 109, 110, 111, 113, 114, 115, 116, 117, 118, 119, 120, 121, 122, 123, 124, 125, 126
workers, 97
workload, 42, 103
workplace, 39
World Health Organization (WHO), viii, 13, 139
worldview, 63
worry, x, 39, 62, 64, 66, 68, 69, 77, 78, 79, 90, 101, 128, 131
writing, 10

Y

yield, 110
young adults, 41